ABOUT THE AUTHORS

MICHAEL FEUERSTEIN, PhD, MPH, is an internationally known clinical psychologist with a specialty in behavioral medicine. For the past decade, he has been on the faculty of Georgetown University Medical Center and Uniformed Services University of Health Sciences as a professor of medical and clinical psychology. He is the editor in chief for the *Journal of Occupational Rehabilitation*. He lives in Maryland.

PATRICIA FINDLEY, DrPH, MSW, LCSW, is a licensed medical social worker and health services researcher specializing in the field of rehabilitation and chronic illnesses. An assistant research professor at Rutgers University's School of Social Work, she formerly was the president of the Spinal Cord Injury Association of Illinois. She lives in New Jersey.

PRAISE FOR *THE CANCER SURVIVOR'S GUIDE:*

"This book is a true learning vehicle on cancer survivorship: it provides step by step measures to mitigate the negatives and provides valuable lessons on how to regain and sustain hope for the future. As a long term and proactive cancer survivor, reading this compelling book gave me pause to think about so many new approaches that I can use in my own survivorship journey."

—NEAL P. LEVITAN, Executive Director, Brain Tumor Society

"*The Cancer Survivor's Guide* provides a unique perspective on strategies for managing the complex and challenging tasks confronting persons diagnosed with cancer. As professionals with expertise in the health-care system, Drs. Feuerstein and Findley take survivors through a step-by-step program that is practical and easy to follow. After reading this book, patients and their families will learn to better navigate the health-care system, manage the stress of diagnosis and treatment, improve their health status and approaches to communicating with their doctors and other support networks, and strategies for achieving a more fulfilling and productive life both during and after their medical treatment has been completed."

—LAWRENCE J. SIEGEL, PhD, ABPP, Dean and Professor, Ferkauf Graduate School of Psychology, Albert Einstein College of Medicine, Yeshiva University

"In *The Cancer Survivor's Guide,* noted health professionals Drs. Michael Feuerstein and Patricia Findley offer a personal and professional prescription for taking control of your life in the face of cancer. This down-to-earth book offers practical how-to advice and inspirational true-life stories to help patients and their families achieve the best possible quality of life."

—WENDY NELSON, PhD, The National Cancer Institute

"*The Cancer Survivor's Guide* resonates through its authenticity, focus, timeliness, and relevance. While cancer occupies a special immediacy among life's wake-up calls, much in this book sheds light throughout the landscape of chronic disease. Dr. Feuerstein and Dr. Findley provide genuine assistance to both patients and healthcare professionals."

—SAM MOON, MD, MPH, Chief of the Division of Occupational and Environmental Medicine, Duke University

"*The Cancer Survivor's Guide* is a wonderful resource for people with cancer. Patients will find the action plans and other tools extremely helpful in their quest for better health care and improvement in the quality of their lives."

—JULIA FAUCETT, PhD, RN, professor and chair
of the department of community health systems at
the University of California in San Francisco

"*The Cancer Survivor's Guide* is forthright, clear, and simple: it provides superb rules for coping with everything from the practical issues of navigating the health care system to how to deal with those demons representing fears of recurrence. I highly recommend this book to cancer survivors and their families."

—JIMMIE C. HOLLAND, MD, Wayne E. Chapman Chair in
Psychiatric Oncology, Memorial Sloan-Kettering Cancer Center

"This inspirational, best of its kind, cutting-edge book provides a roadmap to a healthier and meaningful future following a cancer diagnosis. This enormously helpful guide provides a wealth of life-saving information and tools, providing practical steps that can be taken to ensure the best medical care, to build a strong support team, and to create optimism and hope."

—SUSAN J. BLUMENTHAL, MD, MPA,
Former U.S. Assistant Surgeon General,
Clinical Professor, Georgetown and Tufts Schools of Medicine

"As a father of a child who survived cancer, the indignity of an oncologist having to deal with cancer in my family was how I became aware of survivorship. My experience taught me the importance of comprehensive care of the patient. Drs. Feuerstein and Findley guide the survivor through many of the challenges they face, providing clear information and useful tools to not only maximize the collaboration between patient and physician but to help survivors better manage many of these challenges—which is crucial to successful survivorship."

—STEVEN N. WOLFF, MD, Chairman,
Scientific Advisory Committee, Lance Armstrong Foundation

The
CANCER
SURVIVOR'S
Guide

The CANCER SURVIVOR'S Guide

The Essential Handbook to Life after Cancer

Michael Feuerstein, PhD, MPH,
and Patricia Findley, DrPH, MSW

MARLOWE & COMPANY
NEW YORK

Published by
Marlowe & Company
An Imprint of Avalon Publishing Group Incorporated
245 West 17th Street • 11th floor
New York, NY 10011-5300

A V A L O N
publishing group incorporated

Library of Congress Cataloging-in-Publication Data

Feuerstein, Michael.
The cancer survivor's guide : the essential handbook to life after cancer /
by Michael Feuerstein and Patricia Findley.
p. cm.
Includes bibliographical references.
1. Cancer—Patients—Rehabilitation. 2. Cancer—Psychological aspects.
I. Findley, Patricia. II. Title.
RC262.F48 2006
616.99'403—dc22
2005032452

ISBN: 1-56924-332-8
ISBN-13: 978-1-56924-332-9

9 8 7 6 5 4 3 2 1

Designed by Pauline Neuwirth, Neuwirth & Associates, Inc.
Printed in the United States of America

DISCLAIMER

THE INFORMATION IN this book is intended to help readers make informed decisions about their health and the health of their loved ones. It is not intended to be a substitute for treatment by or the advice and care of a professional health-care provider. While the authors and publisher have endeavored to ensure that the information presented is accurate and up-to-date, they are not responsible for adverse effects or consequences sustained by any persons using this book.

To my family: Shelley, Andrew, Erica, Sara, Umang, and
Kiran, who are my major source of support and joy . . .

To my father, Irving, who is no longer with us but still guides me, and
my mother, Shirley, for instilling and modeling the fighting spirit . . .

To my brother, David, whose love and friendship is so important . . .

MF

To my coauthor, Michael, from whom I've learned and
who has brought me new understanding . . .

To my loving husband and playful friend, Tom,
for never taking me for granted . . .

To my wonderful family: Bob, Gil, Linda, and Jim, who are
always there for me, particularly Mom in heaven . . .

PF

CONTENTS

ACKNOWLEDGMENTS

WHILE I HAVE written acknowledgments for other books over the years, never has this section meant so much to me as now. This is my chance to thank everyone who has helped me over the past three years survive this ordeal so we could pull this together for others.

There were so many. I received the highest-quality care medicine has to offer by the following internist, neurosurgeon, neuro-oncologist, neuro-radiologist, and oncologist: Gary Fisher, MD; Alessandro Olivi, MD; Howard Fine, MD; Shervin Karimpour, MD; and Cheryl Aylesworth, MD. Deanna Glass-Macenka, RN, and Cheryl Royce, RN, neurosurgical and neuro-oncology nurses, were also so helpful during those early days. I was very lucky to have them all as part of my health-care team. Thank you for your scientifically sound, skillful, competent care and human touch.

I am also indebted to my colleagues, friends, and former and current students who have helped me rally my strength so I could keep going and move forward. There are many, but of particular mention are Ian Torrie, MD; Glenn Pransky, MD; Tom Armstrong, PhD; and others at the University of Michigan, Jeff Lackner, PhD; Grant Huang, PhD; Rena Nicholas, PhD; Jenn Hansen, and Lisseth Calvio. My colleagues at the Uniformed Services University of the Health Sciences and Georgetown University Medical Center were also very supportive. I especially would like to mention Neil Grunberg, PhD, who has proven to be a true friend throughout all this. Over the past three years, many others have shown their true colors as colleagues and friends, providing important referral information, encouragement, and understanding. Special thanks to Tracy Sbrocco, PhD; Wendy Law, PhD; Weijo Kopp, PhD; Rich Tannenbaum, PhD; and Meredith Cary, PsyD. Julia Rowland, PhD, director of Cancer Survivorship at the National Cancer Institute at the National Institutes of Health in Bethesda has also generously provided me with her wisdom and support during some tough times. I am very fortunate to know them all.

I chose an ideal professional when I asked Patricia Findley, DrPH, MSW, to collaborate with me on this project. I thought she had the ideal combination of real-world experience in health care along with the critical mind-set of a scientist-practitioner in a field complementary to mine. I thought that together we could create a guide that would address the major challenges of cancer survivorship and provide helpful approaches that survivors could actually use to deal with them. I think I was right. I hope you agree. Working with her on this project has been a joy.

I also want to thank Linda Konner, literary agent, who believed in the premise of this book when others thought it was just "one of those books on cancer." Kylie Foxx saw the usefulness of such a book for survivors and was instrumental in moving this idea to reality. Renée Sedliar, our editor at Avalon Publishing, gave us the guidance we needed to help make this material more user-friendly. I want to thank them all for working with us to get this message across more clearly.

Many consider family members of cancer survivors as also being cancer survivors. This is certainly the case with my family. They have been with me all along. Shelley, my wife, and everyone in my family have shared the initial trauma and the ups and downs of this journey, and it's not over yet. Their love and support has meant so much to me. Shelley has truly been my partner for life. Sharing Sara, Andrew, Erica, Umang, and Kiran's dreams is the biggest joy in my life that keeps me going. Also, as you will see, my youngest daughter, Erica, contributed a passage in the book and I want especially to thank her. Abe, who is no longer with us, Zelda and Pamela Kaplan, Steve and Lisa Criden, and Linda Karch have all been supportive over the years. It means a lot.

I also want to acknowledge the many cancer survivors I have worked with or met while learning to cope with being a cancer survivor myself. Lionel and Sandy Chaiken, who lost their daughter to cancer when she was in her twenties but still keep fighting, and Jeff Shantz, who is an eight-year survivor of a major brain tumor and going strong, are great role models. Jeff continues to be a major source of support for his family and still works full-time as an attorney for the U.S. Department of Justice. They have provided me with wisdom, support, and perspective. I have learned much from their example.

I hope we can help you with the information and tools we have put together.

Michael Feuerstein, PhD, MPH, ABPP
BETHESDA, MARYLAND

I Beat the Odds . . .
Now What?

ON A BEAUTIFUL sunny day in May 2002, I stepped off a curb to cross a busy Washington, D.C., street—and my life as I knew it forever changed. I felt as if I were moving in slow motion. No matter how hard I tried, I couldn't place one foot in front of the other. My legs seemed beyond my control. As I struggled to cross the street, I could hear cars honking. Finally, at the other side of the street, I needed to hold on to a tree. As I tried to regain my composure, an older man commented, "Seems as though you should get a checkup or go see a doctor."

About three minutes later, after I regained control of my legs, I drove home, called my internist, and made an appointment to see him that afternoon. He referred me to a neurologist, who scheduled an MRI for the following week. As I lay in the machine, I reassured myself that everything would be okay. Aside from this small incident of crossing the street, I had not experienced any additional symptoms. "Besides," I told myself, "I'm fit and healthy."

After the MRI, the attending radiologist called me to his office. "The MRI has detected something in your brain. I'm not sure what it is, but it looks serious. Go back to the neurologist who referred you, to go over your results." After hearing his comments, I sat in the waiting room. I now was scared that something might seriously be wrong with me. After a few minutes, I stood up, walked out, and hurried to the neurologist's office at the other end of the building.

The neurologist took a look at the MRI and told me, "It looks like some-thing is growing in the back of your brain, but I don't know exactly what it is," he said. Four MRIs, a full-body CAT scan, many blood tests, open brain surgery, nine physician consultations, and about four weeks later, I learned the true nature of the strange mass growing in my brain. I had a malignant, inoperable brain tumor. My neurosurgeon told me the prognosis was not good. The tumor was a type that had tentacles that could spread to many parts of my brain. He suggested I get my affairs in order. At age fifty-two, I probably had less than a year to live.

I decided to live longer than that. I underwent brain surgery to extract tissue for testing, major radiation to my brain that spanned thirty-three days, and a year of monthly chemotherapy treatments. Now, three years after that initial diagnosis, my MRIs reveal no brain cancer. Despite this happy news, I live with the emotional and physical repercussions of the cancer every day. Certain symptoms, such as fatigue or poor concentration, remind me of the seriousness of my condition. I think of cancer whenever I walk into a hospital, whenever I visit a doctor or see people in wheelchairs, or every fourth month when I go for an MRI.

Not only did I decide to live longer, I also decided to live better, healthier, happier, and more energetically. I decided that getting used to the new normal of reduced energy, memory, and concentration was simply not good enough. I wanted my new normal to closely reflect my old normal. I wanted the energy, mood, and cognitive functions that I had before my treatments.

I realized I had the education and experience and knew to whom to turn to help me realize this goal. As a clinical psychologist with a specialty in behavioral medicine and a degree in public health, and a professor/researcher, I have authored many scientific and medical publications in the areas of pain, rehabilitation, return to work following illness, stress, and, more recently, health services and cancer survivorship. Over the past twenty-five years I have held faculty, administrative, and clinical positions at Stanford Research Institute, McGill University and McGill University Medical Center, University of Florida Health Sciences Center, University of Rochester Medical Center, and recently at the Uniformed Services University of the Health Sciences (federal medical school) in Bethesda, Maryland, and Georgetown University Medical Center in Washington, D.C. My research and clinical work have focused on the area of behavioral medicine/health psychology, helping people (like myself and like you) use modern-day psychology to deal with the challenges of physical health problems. Ironically, over the years I have also run stress-management groups for survivors with many different types of cancer.

I first leaned on my professional background and experience to help me deal with the cancer diagnosis, seeking the best-quality health care and coping with the many challenges I encountered along the way. I continue to use my background to this day, using the skills I've taught so many others to help ensure I communicate effectively with my physicians, talk openly with my family, enlist the support of others when I need it, try not to get too stressed out, and improve my nutritional and lifestyle habits in order to live as healthfully as possible.

Despite my background, however, it wasn't always easy. For some time, after I realized I had beaten the cancer, for example, I lived in limbo. I felt out of touch with my loved ones, my job, and my life in general. Many days I found myself pondering the question, "Now what?" I had expected life *during* cancer to be a challenge. Somehow, I never thought to look forward to life *after* cancer. Although the experience of cancer has changed my life in many positive ways—such as bringing me even closer to my family, allowing me to more easily not let the small things in life bother me, and giving me a greater focus on what is important—survivorship is not without its challenges.

Asking that important question, "Now what?" led me to rediscover the meaning of my life. Leaning on my background as a psychologist, I time and time again used the resources I had, over the years, taught to others with chronic illnesses with great success. You know what? They worked for me, too. I am a more peaceful, happier, healthier person as a result.

As part of my journey as a cancer survivor, I began to find meaning, peace, and satisfaction in helping other survivors who, like myself, found themselves in limbo. I realized that there was no essential guide to help cancer survivors, one that allowed survivors to chart their course for cancer survivorship and answer their own personal "Now what?" That realization and that question eventually led to this book. It's my hope—as well as the hope of my coauthor Patricia—that the tactics you will learn throughout the following pages will do the same for you, allowing you to answer the question, "Now what?" with a specific reaffirmation of life.

THE SCARS OF SURVIVAL

As with anything in life, there are people who go through the cancer experience unscathed. In fact, there are many who have just left it behind them. If you are one of these survivors, I applaud you. You are one of the lucky ones! If you are not, however, you're not alone. Many survivors have deep, bothersome scars. I'm not talking about the physical scars of surgery. I'm talking about those subtle scars. These scars come in the form of memory problems, relationship strains, sexual dysfunction, reproductive concerns, marital discord, work limitations, and financial headaches.

For example, we survivors deal with fear of cancer recurrence on a regular basis. We battle frustrating long-term side effects of treatment, ranging from infertility and impotence to fatigue and concentration problems. Financially, we must find a way to pay for our past and ongoing treatments as well as continue to earn a decent living. Socially, we easily feel out of touch with family, friends, and colleagues who just don't quite understand what it means to be a survivor.

In short, survivorship can be a sad, lonely, scary place. But it doesn't have to be! After getting a clean bill of health from my doctor, I will admit, I wallowed in this sad, lonely, scary place for a while. But, then, as a behavioral health expert, I knew I had to snap out of it, and I did!

To move on, I began using the seven-step program that you will find in this book. Modeled after the United Kingdom's successful Expert Patient program and other self-management approaches to long-term health problems, this seven-step program provides you with a number of very simple tools to beat the challenges of survivorship and move on with your life.

Patients with many different types of chronic illnesses have turned to the United Kingdom's Expert Patient program to help better navigate the health-care system and live life to the fullest. This self-management approach helps people with chronic illnesses learn various skills to more effectively address physical and emotional challenges that accompany their illnesses. In this book, Patricia and I have modified the program to apply specifically to cancer survivors. It provides you with firsthand information on the health-care system in the United States. In addition to learning how to improve the quality of care you receive, you'll also discover many more important tools that aid your survivor journey. From communicating more effectively with your doctor, to finding the motivation to change your eating habits, to addressing lingering posttreatment symptoms, such as pain or fatigue, it's all here. You'll follow a seven-step program that will keep you focused on what's important—your health and quality of life.

You've already heard about what I bring to this project. Now, I'd like to tell you about my coauthor, Dr. Patricia Findley. She has many years of experience as a medical social worker, hospital administrator, and researcher in areas related to health care and disability. She has a master's degree in social work and a doctorate in public health. She surveys hospitals for both the Accreditation Commission for Rehabilitation (CARF) and the Joint Commission on Health Care Organizations. She is currently an assistant research professor at Rutgers University in the School of Social Work and is a fellow in the Institute on Health, Health Care, Aging, and Policy Studies. Her research and publications focus on disability, health disparities, veterans, and the many aspects of the health-care system that impact the care we receive as survivors.

Patricia's desire to collaborate on this book stems from not only her many years of clinical experience, but also from multiple attempts to help her mother better navigate the health-care system. Her mother eventually died at age seventy-two from complications of diabetes. The fragmentation in the health-care system hindered Patricia's mother's ability to fully understand and manage her condition as she was passed from one health-care professional to another. Patricia was amazed at how little individuals working in the health-care system understood the overall system, to help move her mother into the best types of care possible. Her mother did not have the problem-solving skills to act as her own advocate. Patricia tried to advocate and teach, but was frustrated that no single resource was available to help. She also realized how valuable such a resource would have been during her years of clinical work.

With our combined backgrounds, we provide you with the knowledge and skills that are directly important to cancer survivors. In this book, you'll find out what quality medical care is all about. You'll learn how to create and continuously adjust your own medical dream team. You'll also discover how to find and use health information to become a collaborator in your care. Finally, we've provided strategies to help you cope with the physical effects of treatment, living with the uncertainty of long-term survival, resolving stress in general, and maximizing support over the long run.

Many medical studies have shown that components of the program can help you gain more control over symptoms that linger from your treatments as well as help you to effectively deal with the emotions, thoughts, and personal challenges that you face at home and work. When you follow the seven-step program in this book, you will be better able to get the quality health care you need, take responsibility for your health, define your short- and long-term goals, and move toward them.

STEPS TO IMPROVING
YOUR LIFE AFTER CANCER

STEP 1: Make the health-care system work for you. You will learn the ins and outs of the health-care system, and, more importantly, how to put it to work for you. You'll learn how to assess the effectiveness of your health care and health-care team, access low-cost medications, negotiate with your insurance company to cover certain treatments and procedures, and find the right doctors when you need them.

STEP 2: Become a savvy survivor. In this step, you'll sharpen your information-gathering skills. In order to make better decisions about your care and collaborate with your doctors, you'll learn how to find and interpret medical studies. You'll also find out how to understand the pros and cons of different types of complementary medicine and research alternative options on your own. Finally, you'll discover a simple process that will help you to make better decisions about your health care—as well as every other aspect of your life.

STEP 3: Communicate more effectively. Based on what you discovered in steps 1 and 2, you will continue the learning process. This step will help you learn to work with your providers as partners in your long-term health and well-being. You will learn how to communicate more clearly and directly with your words, tone of voice, and body language. As an added bonus, the skills you'll learn in this chapter will help you better communicate your needs in all difficult situations, whether you find yourself asking your supervisor for an accommodation at work or battling with an insurance company over a payment.

STEP 4: Form a strong support team. In this step you learn why you need support and how to get it. A number of helpful hints will help you work on readjusting the level of support you receive through direct communication with loved ones. You'll find out how to ask friends and family to give you support in the way *you* need it. You will explore what spirituality means to you and learn specific ways to practice it, such as meditation. You'll also discover ways to get more support at work. Finally, you will also learn that giving back to others is another aspect of support that survivors often find very helpful.

STEP 5: Find the courage to change. We all want to improve our emotional and physical health, but doing so requires making some changes to our daily routine, changes that aren't always so easy to implement. If you want to exercise more, eat more healthful foods, stop smoking, return to full-time work, and counter cognitive changes that may be reducing your overall effectiveness, this step will arm you with the motivation and knowledge you need to make those changes. These activities can help reduce the symptoms—such as cognitive impairments—that may linger from cancer treatments, prevent age-related health problems such as heart disease, and boost mood and energy levels. In this step, you'll also learn how to speak up for your needs at work—as a result, reducing unneeded stress—as well as better manage the cognitive impairments common among cancer survivors.

STEP 6: See life through more optimistic eyes. This step covers numerous simple approaches to help you better manage stress, depression, and other emotional issues. By using a "stress diary," changing your lifestyle, practicing a simple relaxation exercise, and changing negative thoughts to positive ones, you'll be able to reduce the tension in your days.

STEP 7: Create your future. In this step you will monitor how well you are doing. On a regular basis, you will ask yourself, "How well am I moving toward my goals? Am I doing everything I can? How are my providers doing? Am I managing stress, exercising and adjusting as necessary my levels of social support? How do I feel at work?"

THE REST OF MY STORY—AND YOURS

FOR THREE YEARS since my chemo, the MRIs I receive now every four months have indicated that things are stable—that is, the tumor cannot be seen and cancer cells are not active. I still have a brain tumor, however, and sometimes I just sit quietly and think about what I would do if it came back. I know it can reappear at anytime. When the worry of recurrence strikes me, sometimes I take a walk, read, or just try to relax. Sometimes I talk to my wife or a friend. Sometimes I just immerse myself in my work. Sometimes I tell myself there are lots of things I can do to stay fit and healthy and keep it at bay. Thanks to my ability to remain positive and channel my worry into motivation to improve my health and improve my quality of life, I'm thriving.

This book's "7 Steps to Improving Your Life after Cancer" will help you follow in my footsteps. It's not easy and we will always be working on some aspect of improving our life after cancer. As you move forward through the program, keep in mind that, just as life never seems to move in a straight line, your journey as a cancer survivor won't either. At times, you may proceed forward step by step. Other times, you may want to go back to complete some aspect of an earlier step. So, although we've arranged each step of this program in a logical order that we feel works for most survivors, don't feel pressure to go in order. In each chapter you'll find quizzes that will help you to assess your current situation. These quizzes will help you to quickly see what issues you should address right away—as well as which ones that can safely wait for a while. For now, I encourage you to sit back in your most comfortable chair and just read. Make your way through each chapter, but don't feel compelled to change your life right away. In chapter 7—the last chapter of the book—you'll find the advice you need to figure out what to change first—and how.

So let's get started. In the pages that follow, Patricia and I cover each step, one at a time. With the help of reflective questions, checklists, self-evaluation tools, and specific suggestions, you will be able to experience even better health and a greater quality of life—and finally, once and for all, live the life that is right there in front of you—waiting to be lived.

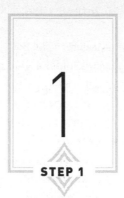

STEP 1

Make the Health-care System
Work for You

THE WORD "SURVIVOR" once only applied to the family members who mourned the loss of someone who had died from cancer. That's no longer the case. Thanks to advances in medicine that have enabled earlier diagnoses and better treatment, more and more people are surviving cancer than ever before. Cancer survivors—people who have finished their primary treatments and are living through repeated recurrences of cancer—total roughly 10 million people in the United States alone!

As survivors we face varied physical, emotional, financial, spiritual, and social challenges. We remain in a period of watching and waiting, wondering if the various symptoms we notice are signs of new tumor growth. We must learn to reconcile ourselves with what oncologists call "the new normal." Cancer and its treatment certainly change us physically. Although we can lessen and possibly even reverse some aftereffects (such as episodic fatigue, mood changes, difficulties with memory and organization, weight gain or loss, inactivity, and pain), others may linger long term. As cancer survivors, we must eat healthfully, exercise, reduce stress, and otherwise live as healthfully as possible both to reduce our risk of a recurrence and of developing such non-cancer-related diseases as diabetes, osteoporosis, and heart disease.

In short, as survivors we need the health-care system more than ever. Although this system works well in diagnosing and treating cancer, it fails miserably in treating the long-term physical, emotional, and cognitive symptoms that many cancer survivors face. For example, after my radiation and chemotherapy, my physicians told me that, other than seeing a neuro-oncologist every three months and undergoing regular MRIs, my treatments were done. I felt grateful that my first-rate cancer care had worked, but I also felt as if this so-called end was really a beginning. I wanted to live as long as possible, reduce the side effects that lingered from cancer treatment, and take as many steps as possible to reduce the risk of a recurrence. So I organized a health-care team to treat me during my survivorship, picking a first-rate internist to manage my general care and seeking out other specialists—including a neurologist–sleep specialist, acupuncturist, massage therapist, otolaryngologist, and a neuropsychologist—as needed. These health professionals helped me with various treatment-induced side effects, including low energy, memory, and fluid buildup in my right ear. They've not only helped me to survive, they've enabled me to *thrive*.

That said, the right doctors, treatments, and medications did not arrive at my doorstep on a silver platter. I had to vigorously *seek them out*. I'm not the first cancer survivor who has done so, and I certainly won't be the last. Many survivors have told me and my coauthor, Patricia, that their initial cancer care was aggressive and comprehensive, with lots of follow-up visits and face-to-face discussions with physicians and other health-care providers. After they finished their major treatments, however, their physicians congratulated them and told them that—other than routine diagnostic tests—they needed no further care. These survivors felt as if they were in limbo, with no clear path to follow. Over the years Patricia and I have helped these survivors to develop a health-care plan for their life after cancer, one that helped them to locate the best doctors so they could get the treatments, tests, and medications they need and address their emotional and lifestyle needs.

You can benefit from a similar plan. Now that you've concluded your major treatments, do you still have a team of physicians in place to help you manage physical and emotional symptoms that linger from your initial cancer battle? Do you have a plan for staying healthy and improving the quality of your life, such as relationships with those you care about, managing stress at work and home, pain, or getting the support you need to carry on? If you answered yes to both questions, that's wonderful! I congratulate you, because you are in the minority. Still I urge you to read on, because you will no doubt find some strategies in this chapter that can help you even more.

What if you answered no to one or both of those questions? Then, read on. You deserve the best care possible at the time when you need it. You will face many challenges. To successfully deal with those challenges, you will need a top-notch health-care team in place. To form this team, you first, however, need a realistic perspective of health care in America. In this chapter, that's exactly what you'll find. You'll learn what you—as a cancer survivor—need to know to get the best quality of care possible to stay healthy, prevent a recurrence, and reduce treatment-induced symptoms. After reading this chapter, you will better understand the resources available to you, how to best use them, and how to avoid the many pitfalls of modern day medicine.

The information you will find in this chapter—and throughout this book—will help you map out your path to better health, finally defining clearly and definitively just what you as a survivor need to do to continue to survive with the best quality of life possible. To get the most out of the health-care system as a survivor, you must *work* the system. It shouldn't be this way, but it is, and no amount of complaining will change it.

You've probably read in many self-help books and articles that you must remain optimistic, that optimism sets the stage for survival. That's true to a point. You also must remain *realistic*. Cancer is a serious life-threatening illness. Yes, remain optimistic about your health; you've survived

> ## *Survivor Stat*
>
> CANCER SURVIVORS are less likely than the general population to receive recommended care for their non-cancer-related chronic health-care problems, such as diabetes, heart disease, or recommended preventive health-care services.

and will continue to do so. But also remain realistic. Don't ignore symptoms such as fatigue, headaches, feelings of depression, weight gain, and insomnia—and don't let your doctor ignore them, either. Don't sit back and let your doctor drive your health. Become informed. Ask questions. Become part of your health-care team. Doing so will help ensure that you live longer and better!

This realistic optimism starts with the health-care system. To work it, you must understand it. You must first know what quality health care is, to have a measuring stick to gauge whether you are getting it. Then, once you see how your care measures up, you'll need to do something about it. Don't simply count on the right things happening. Make them happen!

THE STATE OF HEALTH CARE

AS PART OF my course work to earn a master's in public health, I studied the delivery of health care in the United States and around the world. Patricia did similar research when she earned her doctorate in the scientific study of health care. Patricia and I have spent many years working as administrators of health care in medical centers, rehabilitation facilities, and hospitals. We have also worked on national teams that accredit these institutions.

That research and personal experience has given us an inside look at how the health-care system in the United States works—or doesn't work. Not only is health care in our country a privilege; quality health care can be a gamble. While the United States tops the charts for how much citizens and the government spend on health care, we as citizens experience more disease than do citizens of other industrialized countries.

At its best, the U.S. health-care system is a fragmented hodgepodge of providers, laws, policies, drug companies, government-funded health care (such as Veteran's Administration, Medicare, and Medicaid programs), and privately funded health care (insurance companies). It is really *not* a system at all. Here's a closer look at what you're up against.

Patient overload: The average doctor spends roughly seven minutes with each patient. This generally is not enough time to address the complex problems cancer survivors experience.

Conflicts among providers and insurance carriers: One in three doctors report they do not suggest potentially effective health-care services if a patient's insurance will not cover it.

Lack of follow-up care: Many patients don't get the most effective and up-to-date treatment. In fact, research shows that patients in the United States receive only half the care recommended by medical evidence. This is especially true for preventative care.

Medical errors: According to the Institute of Medicine (IOM), medical errors cause more deaths each year than do breast cancer, car accidents, and AIDS combined! According to the IOM, many of these errors could be prevented with proper staffing.

Inconsistent quality control: Each physician has different motivations, skills, and knowledge. While some certainly go well beyond the call of duty, others do not recommend routine health checks and physicals, forcing you to stay on top of these important preventative health needs.

Avoiding Medical Errors

WATCH OUT FOR these medical errors:

Error: Failure to follow up on tests or monitoring programs
Prevent it by: Making sure you follow up by calling your primary care doctor or specialist's office. You need those results to find out what, if anything, needs to be done next.

Error: Prescribing the wrong type or amount of medication
Prevent it by: Researching on the internet to make certain the medication and dose is right for you. You can also talk with the nurse or call your local pharmacy. Pharmacists are willing to discuss your medication with you. Also monitor for any side effects that may indicate the dosage needs to be adjusted.

Error: Failure to suggest known ways to prevent common problems cancer survivors encounter
Prevent it by: Staying on top of research completed on cancer survivors and talking to other cancer survivors about their treatment

Error: Failure to suggest a test that may have helped
Prevent it by: Checking to see what tests are recommended by evidence-based guidelines for your specific situation. During every visit, ask your doctor, "Is there anything more that can help this particular situation?"

Error: Suggesting the wrong type of care
Prevent it by: Consulting clinical practice guidelines for the problem and comparing them to your treatment.

> **Error:** Failure to keep you informed of your situation
> **Prevent it by:** Asking your doctor about his or her recommenda-
> tions, explaining that you want to know the evidence behind his or
> her advice. Also, talk with a nurse in the office and, if that doesn't
> work, get a new doctor.

It's really a mess. Although many factors—including your income and insurance—influence the care you receive, the most important of all of the factors that influence your care is you. You must learn how to manage this system to ensure you'll thrive. Although less than perfect, the U.S. health-care system does not *have to* be a source of frustration. You can maximize its potential. Before you do so, however, you must understand how it works.

According to the Institute of Medicine, quality health care means:

1. You can obtain care when you need it, in many forms (face to face, Internet, telephone, from different providers).
2. Your care is customized based on your needs and values.
3. You have a high degree of control over your health care and health-care decisions. Your doctors support your desire to share decision-making.
4. You feel comfortable sharing information with your providers, who freely communicate all information about diagnoses, tests, and treatments.
5. You receive care based on the best available scientific evidence.
6. You are free from errors of omission, or care that is wrong given your current situation.
7. You have the information you need to make reasonable decisions about which health plan, hospital, clinical practice, or alternative treatment to use.
8. Your doctor or health-care group anticipates your health needs instead of just reacting to illness.
9. You don't wait for weeks or months for an appointment with a specialist or for an important test. You also don't wait for hours in the waiting room.
10. All your providers, hospitals, and/or clinics communicate and work with one another for your care. They agree that care for someone with cancer never ends.

How does your care measure up? Use the following checklist, Getting the Best Possible Care, to assess your current level of care. Then, read on to find out how to improve the care you receive—no matter how good or bad your current situation.

Getting the Best Possible Care

Quality health care stems from three factors: *access, cost,* and *quality providers.* You must have access to skilled physicians, correct and accurate tests and interpretations, and well-supported treatments, and be able to pay for them. All three areas work together. To see how your care measures up for each area, check yes or no for each of the following questions. After each section, total up the number of no responses.

	AREA I: ACCESS TO CARE		
	ACCESS	**Y**	**N**
1	I have a doctor I see on a regular basis.		
2	I can see my doctor whenever I need.		
3	When my doctor does not have the knowledge or skills to help me, he or she tells me the type of specialist I need for my specific problem.		
4	When my doctor recommends a procedure or prescribes a medication, he or she explains why and the explanation seems to make sense.		
5	My doctor coordinates my care with other doctors.		
6	My doctor asks me whether I've made appointments to see specialists or undergo testing that he or she has recommended to me in the past. My doctor also keeps track of these test results and information from these specialists about my health.		
7	The specialists I see follow up with me and my doctor.		
8	I follow up with my doctor on a problem if I still have concerns, such as if I think a medication is not working.		
9	My health insurance plan allows me to see the specialists I need.		
10	When I need a test or a procedure, the hospital or clinic schedules me in a timely manner.		
	Total		

AREA II: QUALITY		
QUALITY	**Y**	**N**
1	I know what clinical practice guidelines (CPGs) say about the tests and treatments available for my specific problem.		
2	I have a copy of the CPG for health problems I am trying to fix at the moment.		
3	I can talk to my doctor about these treatment guidelines.		
4	My doctor spends enough time with me to fully understand and treat all the problems I wish to address.		
5	I can tell my doctor all my concerns.		
6	I use other types of doctors or practitioners when I need them, such as alternative medicine experts, physical therapists, psychologists, or social workers.		
7	My doctor follows up on my care over the long run.		
8	My doctor helps me stay healthy.		
9	The staff at hospitals and clinics where I receive my care treat me like a patient and a person, and not a number.		
10	My doctors, hospitals, and clinics have good reputations.		
	Total		

AREA III: COST		
COST	**Y**	**N**
1	My health insurance covers most of my care.		
2	I have health insurance.		
3	I have enough money to pay for fitness or nutritional recommendations.		
4	I can afford to have my eyes and teeth checked regularly.		
5	I can afford to buy the medication my doctor recommends.		
6	I can afford to buy special medical equipment or supplies when my doctor recommends them.		
7	The cost of care does not prevent me from getting the care I need, such as the cost of seeing a specialist.		
8	I can afford food or clothing, even though I need to pay doctors' bills.		

9	My insurance covers health screenings (e.g., blood tests to check cholesterol levels, diabetes checks, repeat physicals or screenings).		
10	I do not skip recommended treatments (e.g., filling medications or going to physical therapy) because I know insurance or I can pay for them.		
	Total		

Place your totals in the chart below. For example, if you had 7 no answers in the access section, you would then multiply 7 by 10, and get 70 percent.

AREAS	NUMBER OF NO'S	MULTIPLY BY 10	PERCENTAGE
Access			
Quality			
Cost			

Now place an *x* on the Health-care Barriers chart, next to the percentages you just determined. In other words, if you had seven no answers in the access section, five no answers in the quality section, and two no answers in the cost section, you'd place an *x* next to 70, 50, and 20, as shown in the sample grid. This means there are seven things you need to improve in your ability to get medical help when you need it, five things

		Sample Grid					Insert Your Own Scores		
		HEALTH-CARE BARRIERS					**HEALTH-CARE BARRIERS**		
		ACCESS	QUALITY	COST			ACCESS	QUALITY	COST
NEED FOR CHANGE	100				**NEED FOR CHANGE**	100			
	90					90			
	80					80			
	70	X				70			
	60					60			
	50		X			50			
	40					40			
	30					30			
	20			X		20			
	10					10			
	0					0			

to improve in terms of quality, and just two things to improve under cost. You eventually want to lower your percentage to 0 percent in each area, meaning you have worked to remove all barriers.

ASSEMBLE YOUR DREAM TEAM

DOCTORS, NURSES, PHARMACISTS, and other professionals make up your health-care team. For many survivors, these team members remain the same from treatment through survival, but not always. If your physicians and other providers specialize in cancer treatment and not in cancer survival—and tell you as much—you may need to shop around for new team members.

The most important person on your health-care team is your oncologist, internist, or primary care physician who sees you regularly and coordinates your care among all of the other team members you see. According to one study, cancer survivors who regularly consulted with a primary care physician or an oncologist received the health care they needed to treat symptoms and monitor their cancer more often than did survivors who did not have a regular doctor. Whether you see an oncologist, family doctor, or internist, one fact remains clear: you must continue to see *someone* regularly.

As a survivor, you need a doctor who you can see for any problem and who coordinates your care, communicating with the rest of your care team and ensuring that all of the health-care professionals who treat you know about your care, health, and well-being. This physician will help you maintain your health and speed your recovery following a short-term illness. It is not enough to simply go to a doctor recommended to you by a friend or family member. As a cancer survivor, you need to critically judge your providers in the same way you would judge a car repair shop.

To find the right person for this all-important role, you'll first want to evaluate your current oncologist, family doctor, or internist. Use the checklist Evaluate Your Relationship with Your Provider to complete this evaluation. In addition to your results from this checklist, consider your actual health as well. You may decide not to rock the boat if blood tests, x-rays, MRIs, CAT scans, and other diagnostic tests indicate that your health seems to be improving or stable.

Evaluate Your Relationship with Your Provider

COMPLETE THIS CHECKLIST for all your providers. Not every provider will have all of these characteristics, but your major health providers should have most of them.

Circle a Yes or No in response to each of the following questions:

1. Do you feel your doctor uses the latest, most up-to-date care?　　Yes　No
2. Does your doctor help you coordinate care with all your providers?　　Yes　No
3. Do you feel your doctor understands/listens you?　　Yes　No
4. Does your doctor seem to care about you in an emotional sense?　　Yes　No
5. Do you feel confident about your doctor's medical knowledge?　　Yes　No
6. Are you treated with respect in the doctor's office?　　Yes　No
7. Are you able to bring up concerns without feeling as if you are taking too much of your doctor's time?　　Yes　No
8. Do you feel that your doctor can admit mistakes if they occur?　　Yes　No
9. Are you comfortable in the office environment?　　Yes　No
10. Would you refer a friend or family member to your doctor?　　Yes　No

Add up the total Yes and No items circled.
Total Yes_____ Total No_____

If you have **9 to 10** yes responses, congratulations! You seem to have found a provider with whom you are comfortable to help manage your survivorship.

If you have **6 to 8** yes responses, you may want to discuss your concerns with your provider and think about finding a new one.

If you have **6 or fewer** yes responses, consider finding a new provider. Your confidence and ability to work with your providers is key in your successful survivorship.

If you decide you and your doctor could do better, have an honest discussion with him or her. Often, with open and honest communication, you can turn many of these problems around, especially regarding the need for a new referral to a specialist or the need to initiate a conversation regarding some other aspect of your care. Resist the urge to avoid this conversation. You want to stay as healthy as possible, and these doctors can help make that happen.

However, if communication doesn't work, it's time to go doctor shopping. Most important, make sure you choose a doctor who is familiar with and who follows evidence-based clinical practice guidelines. These guidelines give providers and patients a road map of the most effective care, based on the best available research. Evidence-based clinical practice guidelines dictate how medicine can best evaluate and treat many clinical problems, such as various types of cancer, high blood pressure, diabetes, pain, or fatigue. Generated by health-care professionals with experience treating these specific problems, these guidelines are based on studies and clinical experience.

The use of guidelines has helped make care more consistent from provider to provider; however, some doctors choose not follow them. Such doctors complain these guidelines represent "cookbook" medicine or are not useful for all patients with a particular condition. It's true that medicine is both an art and a science, but these guidelines—when thoughtfully considered by you and your physician—help improve outcomes. Ask potential physicians how they arrive at their recommendations. Do they base their recommendations, at least in part, on an evidence-based guideline and on the latest scientific evidence? They should.

In addition to looking for a physician who is in step with the latest research, look for a physician with the following qualities:

Someone who knows medicine: Many Web sites will help you determine the competency of your physicians. One of these sites, Health-Grades.com (www.healthgrades.com) rates physicians, but charges you for that information. The American Medical Association (www .ama-assn.org) provides similar information, as do individual state medical associations. Through these organizations, you can find out if a doctor is licensed, his or her specialty areas, where he or she attended medical school, and the year he or she graduated. Also, each state publishes a list of actively licensed physicians as well as those whose licenses have been suspended. You can access many of those reports on the state Web sites for the Department of Professional Regulation.

Understanding Evidence-Based Guidelines

EVIDENCE-BASED GUIDELINES CAN help you ensure that the test or treatment for your specific problem is on track with the best scientific evidence. While medical evidence grows faster than these guidelines can be revised and updated, they do provide a good framework for state-of-the-art care, and support your realistic optimism about the basic elements of your actual care and what to expect from them in terms of usefulness and clinical effects or their outcome. For example, if an expert guideline is available for you for a problem you have, it can serve as your roadmap in your journey to get help with the problem. Many, but not all, doctors rely on these guidelines. Many guidelines have been made available to patients on the following Web sites:

- **www.guideline.gov**—The national guideline clearinghouse agency for health-care research and quality
- **www.hsl.mcmaster.ca/ebm**—McMaster University Health Sciences Library
- **www.qmo.amedd.army.mil**—The U.S. Army's MEDCOM Quality Management Office; click on practice guidelines
- **www.ahrq.gov**—The U.S. Agency for Health Care Research and Quality
- **www.nccn.org**—National Comprehensive Cancer Network

Every state has its own rules for regulation; although they are fairly similar, you will need to locate the correct one for your state.

Someone who knows cancer and cancer survival: Consult the support services at your local cancer centers or closest academic medical center. These services offer experts in medical care of cancer survivors, psychology, social work, nutrition, pastoral care, health education, and nursing. Although these integrative programs follow long-term survivors, they are not very common. If you don't live near a cancer center, ask other survivors to recommend physicians to you. Go to the American Cancer Society's cancer survivor discussion

boards (www.acscsn.org) to chat with other survivors about helpful physicians, as well as the Lance Armstrong Foundation at www
.livestrong.org.

Someone who follows up: Look for a physician who suggests preventive health care on some regular basis such as cholesterol screenings, bone scans, blood sugar tests, physicals, and screenings for other cancers. To find out what tests you need when, consult the U.S. Preventive Services Task Force or the Agency for Healthcare Research and Quality (www.ahrq.gov). Once at the Web site, look into the consumer health section to find layman's language versions of clinical practice guidelines on a variety of topics and conditions. If possible, before choosing a doctor, ask whether he or she follows these guidelines.

Someone who works with you: Look for a doctor who is willing to serve as a collaborative partner in your care and not for someone who always wants to tell you what to do. You'll have many choices during your survival. You want a doctor who lays out the pros and cons, and helps you arrive at a confident decision.

Round Out Your Team with Specialists

In addition to your lead physician, you'll also supplement your health-care team with other members as needed. Many of these team members will be specialists who can help you with various treatment-related symptoms that many general physicians are not trained to address.

For example, after radiation treatment, I could not hear well in my right ear. I found it more and more difficult to make out what other people were saying. My oncologist could not pinpoint the problem and suggested I see an ear, nose, and throat (ENT) doctor. I did. This specialist was able to diagnose fluid behind my eardrum that had built up from the radiation. This specialist drained the fluid, and my hearing improved.

The ear, nose, and throat physician is just one of many specialists I've seen during the past two years since my major treatments have ended. Of course it would be nice to have a one-stop shop of a physician who could treat every symptom, but this just isn't the case.

Physicians usually have one of two types of degrees; they are either an MD (medical doctor) or a DO (doctor of osteopathy). Basically, these degrees are very similar. Both kinds of doctors are licensed medical professionals. Years ago, medical schools trained these physicians differently. For example, DOs were trained to view patients in a very holistic manner, considering both home and work environments. However, today the training between the two is pretty much the same.

All physicians have general core training, but then they go on to complete additional course work, training, and/or residencies to gain a specialty. Specialists usually become "board certified" in their specialty area. This means that they complete the additional training requirements ("hands on," clinical, and book learning) and take an exam to meet the requirements of the specialty board. Make sure your physician specialists are board certificated in their area of specialty, as these providers went an extra step to be evaluated by their peers in terms of knowledge and, often, skills.

In addition to medical doctors and doctors of osteopathy, you also may need to consult a number of nonphysician specialists. Many of these experts—such as physician's assistants and nurse practitioners—can spend more time with you, describing your physician's diagnoses and treatment in more detail, and helping you work around the complexities that are often found in certain aspects of health care.

To know what type of specialist to add to your health-care team—and when—consult the list of health-care providers and their specialties, Specialists Who Can Round Out Your Team, on pages 15–16. Although not comprehensive, the list will give you ideas about specialists you may need to add to your team. In addition to consulting that list, ask your primary doctor for recommendations.

SPECIALISTS WHO CAN ROUND OUT YOUR TEAM	
PHYSICIAN SPECIALIST	**WHAT THEY DO**
Endocrinologist	A physician who has completed several years of training in the field of endocrinology, the study of hormones and the internal glands, such as the thyroid and pancreas.
Reproductive Endocrinologist	A physician who specializes in reproductive medicine. These specialists are sometimes referred to as "fertility specialists."
Nephrologist	A physician who has been educated and trained in kidney diseases, kidney transplantation, and dialysis therapy

continued

PHYSICIAN SPECIALIST	WHAT THEY DO
Neurologist	A physician who has trained in the diagnosis and treatment of nervous system disorders, including diseases of the brain, spinal cord, nerves, and muscles.
Neuro-oncologist	A physician who specializes in treating patients with brain tumors, and/or the consequences of cancer upon the nervous system. The physician may be a trained neurologist, oncologist, or neurosurgeon.
Neuroradiologist	A radiologist who specializes in the use of radioactive substances, x-rays, and scanning devices for the diagnosis and, possibly, treatment of diseases of the brain and other components of the nervous system.
Neurosurgeon	A physician trained in surgery of the nervous system.
Oncologist	A physician who specializes in treating cancer.
Pain Specialist	These anesthesiologists, neurologists, physical medicine specialists, family practitioners, neurosurgeons, orthopeadic surgeons, and orthopeadists are knowledgeable in the area of pain evaluation and its medical treatment. There are also nonphysicians who play an important role is helping to manage persistent pain such as health psychologists, physical therapists, occupational therapists, and acupuncturists. You can look into this at the American Pain Society (www.ampainsoc .org or call 1-847-375-4715) or the International Society for the Study of Pain (www.iasp-pain.org or call. 1-206-547-6409).
Pathologist	A physician trained in the nature, cause, process, and effects of disease. Pathologists examine samples of tissue removed during surgery to determine an exact diagnosis.
Radiologist	A physician trained in the use of radioactive substances, x-rays, and other imaging techniques to arrive at a diagnosis.

NONPHYSICIAN SPECIALISTS	WHAT THEY DO
Case Manager/ Case Coordinator	This person may help you to work with your insurance company or help you get through the current hospitalization and get back into your home, school, and/or job. Frequently, a nurse or a social worker fills this role.
Behavioral Health Specialists	These clinical psychologists and neuropsychologists specialize in the psychological and behavioral aspects of medical illness. He or she can help you with your attitude and mood and teach you ways to reduce stress and pain; improve your communication and coping skills; and help you with health behavior changes, such as weight loss, smoking, taking medication. A neuropsychologist can help you better understand and deal with the reasons why you are having problems with memory, attention, learning, and other functions influenced by the brain.
Chiropractors	These health professionals treat patients whose health problems are associated with the body's muscular, nervous, and skeletal systems, particularly the spine. Chiropractors believe that these systems should work together without imbalance; otherwise, the person becomes susceptible to disease. The chiropractic approach to health care is holistic, stressing the patient's overall health and wellness. Chiropractors do not prescribe medications; rather, they provide natural, drugless, nonsurgical treatments that rely on the body's own natural ability to heal. These practitioners have limited licenses to practice spinal manipulation, and unlike the MDs and the DOs, they are not allowed to admit patients to a hospital or perform surgery.

Take a Breather

We have covered a lot of material! It's okay to step back for a moment and think about what you've read and what you're going through. This may be the time to set this book down and take a walk or talk to a friend. We'll start up again when you are ready.

KNOW THE PHARMACEUTICAL INDUSTRY

THANKS TO NEW medications, more people are surviving cancer than ever before. Indeed, a group of new drugs now respond specifically to the biological mechanisms or pathways of cancer. These new medications also help minimize the impact of surgery.

Before you write a thank you note to one of your favorite drug companies, however, consider the following:

- The Food and Drug Administration (FDA) has come under scrutiny in recent years for hastily approving some medications without fully considering their side effects. Why would this happen? First, drug companies pay the FDA user fees to speed up drug approvals. Second, according to a *USA Today* investigation, more than half of the experts hired to advise the FDA about the safety and effectiveness of drugs have close financial relationships with the pharmaceutical industry. These financial conflicts were cited as a top reason that the FDA approved the drug Vioxx, later removed from the market after studies revealed it raised risk for heart attack and stroke.
- The top U.S. drug makers spend 2.5 times as much money on marketing and administration as they do on research. These sophisticated ads urge you to visit your doctor to ask about this or that medication for all types of symptoms.
- About 75 percent of new drugs approved by the FDA are less effective than current drugs already on the market. As long as they're more effective than a placebo, the FDA allows them onto the market.

You, of course, can't solve the nation's drug problems on your own, but you can take effective steps to make sure you take only the most effective medications that pose the fewest side effects possible. Do the following:

Pay attention to the list of side effects in drug ads. Drug companies are required by law to list the side effects of their medications in their advertisements. If you see an ad for a drug that you think might be helpful, write down the name of the drug, its benefits, and its side effects. Take this note with you the next time you visit your doctor and ask your doctor for his or her advice. If you decide to take the medication, use the monitoring form on page 20, Is My Medication Working? to keep track of side effects you experience and how effectively the medication manages your symptoms. Discuss your results with your doctor every few months.

Look into ways to reduce your medication bill. Many pharmaceutical companies offer free and reduced cost drugs to people in need. For example, GalxoSmithKline offers a 30 to 40 percent discount to seniors, those with disabilities, and Medicare beneficiaries with annual incomes below $30,000 to $40,000, depending on marital status. Merck and Pfizer offer similar programs. Determine which manufactures the medications you need, call the company's customer service number, and ask how to get enrolled in a patient assistance program. Check out the Web site for NeedyMeds.com (www. needymeds.com). It lists every pharmaceutical company's charity drug program, along with contact information, application forms, and procedures to follow. Also check out the Web site www.themedicineprogram. com. This nonprofit program will help you to complete forms and apply for reduced cost or free medications, charging you only $5 per prescription.

Purchase mail-order drugs from a reputable company. Mail-order pharmacies can save you money, but sometimes you get what you pay for, especially if these pharmacies are overseas! According to the Food and Drug Administration, nearly 90 percent of the imported mail-order drugs stopped at the borders by government agents were potentially dangerous or illegal. They included drugs that had been pulled from the U.S. market, animal drugs never approved for human use, counterfeit drugs, and drugs with dangerous side effects.

> ### *Survivor Stat*
>
> Pʜᴀʀᴍᴀᴄᴇᴜᴛɪᴄᴀʟ ɪɴᴅᴜꜱ-ᴛʀʏ spending on direct-to-consumer advertising increased from $46.6 million in 1990 to approximately $1 billion in 1997. These fancy ads work! They make you want these meds—stat. Trust your physician to make the final call of the medications you need. We get a lot of marketing messages, but your physicians have the education and training to help you see the truth in advertising.

In addition to those potential problems, heat can reduce the effectiveness of some types of medications. Some reputable mail-order pharmacies, such as Medco, circumvent this issue by packaging heat-sensitive medications on dry ice. If you use a mail-order pharmacy, always check the labels on your medications to see how they should be stored. If the medicine should be refrigerated and the company mailed it in a regular envelope, it's time to switch mail-order pharmacies!

Use the same pharmacy to fill all of your prescriptions. Your pharmacy can watch out for common drug interactions that your team of health providers may not catch. For example, your primary care doctor might prescribe a drug to treat one symptom and a specialist might prescribe a drug to treat a completely different symptom. If the doctors don't communicate—and they often don't—you may end up taking two drugs that counteract or negatively interact with one another!

KNOW THE INSURANCE INDUSTRY

ALTHOUGH HAVING INSURANCE does not guarantee you access to quality health care these days, it certainly helps. Indeed, in a recent survey, one in three doctors admitted they would not mention effective treatments to patients if insurance did not cover those treatments. Another study, published in the *New England Journal of Medicine,* found that only half of the care recommended by a physician was ever covered by insurance companies.

Even if you have insurance as a cancer survivor, it's not a guarantee that you will continue to receive the health care you need. If you have private insurance and switch from one provider to another, for example, you

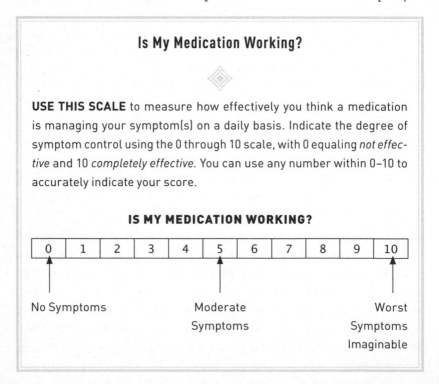

Is My Medication Working?

USE THIS SCALE to measure how effectively you think a medication is managing your symptom(s) on a daily basis. Indicate the degree of symptom control using the 0 through 10 scale, with 0 equaling *not effective* and 10 *completely effective.* You can use any number within 0–10 to accurately indicate your score.

IS MY MEDICATION WORKING?

0	1	2	3	4	5	6	7	8	9	10

No Symptoms   Moderate   Worst
                     Symptoms   Symptoms
                                       Imaginable

DATE	TIME	PAIN RATING	MEDICATION	EFFECTIVENESS RATING	SIDE EFFECTS FROM MEDICATION
Sample Entry: October 14	7am	7	Ibuprofen	3	stomach upset, rash, constipation

may have to go through a process called *medical underwriting*. During this process, the prospective insurance company looks at your health history and medical records, and then decides whether it will cover you and, if so, at what rate. Sometimes such insurers charge hefty premiums for cancer survivors or will not cover related problems for a certain period of time because they deem cancer a "preexisting condition." In this case, the health insurance plan may cover other medical care, but you will have to pay out-of-pocket for follow-up care related to your cancer and cancer treatment.

According to the Health Insurance Portability and Accountability Act of 1996 (HIPPA), a preexisting condition exclusion must relate to a condition for which medical advice, diagnosis, care, or treatment was recommended or received during the six-month period prior to an individual's enrollment date for the insurance. The preexisting condition exclusion may not last for more than twelve months (eighteen for late enrollees) after an individual's enrollment date; and this twelve-month period must be reduced by the number of days of your previous insurance coverage, excluding coverage before any break in coverage of sixty-three days or more. Although this is the law, you'll need to check with potential insurance companies to clarify individual situations.

The bottom line: if you have insurance that is acceptable and you can stay on it, do so. Why rock the boat? If you change insurance carriers, be cautious and never go longer than sixty-three days without insurance! (It will decrease your ability to be covered again.) If you are shopping for insurance, you generally have the following options:

- A group employer-sponsored plan if you work for a large company
- An individual, private insurance plan if you are self-employed
- A government program, such as Medicare or Medicaid if you meet specific income, age, or disability requirements, (Medicaid eligibility varies state to state, so consult Appendix A for the contact information for these programs), or a Veteran's Administration plan if you served in the military

Health insurance plans are generally set up one of two ways. One is called a Health Maintenance Organization (HMO). These plans provide a network of doctors, other health-care professionals, hospitals, laboratories, and other related services. You usually have to select from providers within your HMO's network, for the insurer to cover your care. The second is a Preferred Provider Organization (PPO). This type of health plan also provides a network of doctors, but the network is larger than an HMO, and you can go to any of the doctors, health-care professionals, and hospitals within that plan. You usually do not need a referral to go to a specialist. However, the premiums for these plans are usually more expensive.

If you change employers, or if you work for a large employer with coverage options, you may want to carefully consider changing your insurer during open season for doing so. To pick the right plan for you, do the following:

1. Review the specific services that the insurance covers and note any that are *not* covered.
2. Find out how much the premiums cost.
3. Determine the deductible amounts.
4. Find out what you will pay out-of-pocket for covered services.
5. Check to see which providers you are allowed to use under the policy, and whether your physicians are included.

No matter what type of insurance you have, you most likely will need to confront your carrier at some point over what's covered and what's not covered. If you sit back and do nothing, your insurance policy will drive your health care, influencing the care you receive—or don't receive—and your overall health. With some dogged advocacy on your part, however, you can turn this around.

To do so, you must understand the logic behind your insurance company's policies. To try to convince the company to cover a treatment, you must know your policy inside and out. Get a copy from the human resources representative at your employer. Read the fine print that comes with your policy to learn about your coverage and how to access your benefits. For help in understanding your policy, look for a toll-free number or a Web address on your insurance card, premium statements, or explanation of benefits pages. Consult a representative at your insurance company or your providers' business offices for help in understanding what your policy covers.

It is important for you to be an informed policyholder. If a treatment is refused for coverage, it is for one of three reasons: (1) it's not "within the scope of the policy," or (2) it's not "medically necessary," or (3) it's "experimental." So what do these mean?

If the treatment is not "within the scope of your policy," it means that it is not a covered benefit for all policyholders, regardless of circumstance. When policies are written, the employer is deciding what to include based on how much they want to pay to provide coverage for their employees. Sometimes under special circumstances, you can work with your employer's benefit office and their insurance contact to try to get something covered. This takes patience, documentation of need from the physician, and your good communication skills. Keep your cool, your optimism, and follow the advice of the employer in the process. One time, Patricia was able to get extended benefits for a patient. The patient was well liked by his employer and the personal contact by the patient to the employer from the hospital, facilitated by Patricia, helped increase the employer's willingness to go to bat for him with the insurance company. In the end, the patient got all the coverage he needed. Although these types of requests are a long-shot, it does not hurt to try.

With services that are deemed "not medically necessary," you need to be aware that this can mean that the insurance company, based on its practices and policies, does not cover the service or procedure that your doctors are requesting for you. It can also mean that insufficient information regarding your situation was included with the request to justify the need for the service. Either way, more information is essential. You should contact both your insurance company and your health-care provider to gather information on what is needed to show the insurance company your need and to let your health-care provider know what is necessary. If in the end, the service is still considered not medically necessary, you need to continue to work with your health-care provider to see if there is another treatment that may help you.

Finally, to evaluate whether a treatment is "experimental" most insurance companies look to the Blue Cross and Blue Shield Association's criteria to determine if a treatment is experimental. A treatment is experimental if it does *not* meet all five of these criteria:

1. It has approval of the appropriate governmental regulatory body (such as the FDA).
2. Scientific research has shown that the treatment affects health.
3. The treatment improves health.
4. The treatment must be as helpful as other known treatments.
5. The benefits of the treatment must be shown to work outside of research projects.

Your doctor can tell you whether the treatment he or she is recommending, or the treatment you've read about or interested in, is experimental or not. You will also be able to tell if something is experimental by the informed consent documents that you will be asked to sign before the procedures (see Know the Laws on page 29 for more about informed consent). These forms will explain to you whether a treatment will not be covered by your insurance, because you will be expected to pay for it. If these forms seem overwhelming to read, ask your doctor if you can take them home rather than signing on the spot. Or, ask if you can see the forms fifteen minutes before your scheduled treatment time, so you have time to

Alternative Ways to Pay for Treatments

IF YOUR INSURER won't pay for a test or treatment, consider the following additional ways to pay for treatments.

If you have served in the military, consult the Veterans Administration (VA). The VA provides a comprehensive health-care program at no cost, or low cost to qualified veterans. To determine your eligibility, contact the Department of Veterans Affairs (see Appendix A). If you are active duty or retired military, TRICARE Prime, a comprehensive health-care program, will insure you and your dependents (see Appendix A for contact information).

Medicaid, the state health insurance plan, may be an option, but to qualify for this type of insurance, you must have a very low income, and in most states, have a disability. Check with your state's Medicaid agency or your medical social worker to learn if you are a likely candidate.

Negotiate with hospitals or providers for free or reduced-cost care. Many doctors and hospitals provide what is called "charity care." Hospitals actually plan for such care in their annual budget and each year are prepared to "write off" or give away a certain amount of care for free. The 1999 Medicare Payment Advisory Committee found that hospitals had $20.8 billion in uncompensated care. Also, a 1994 survey by the American Medical Association's Socioeconomic Monitoring System found that 67.7 percent of doctors offered either free or reduced-price care and spent an average of 7.2 hours a week delivering charity care. In addition to free care, many physicians have access to free or reduced-price medications that they get either through drug companies or state programs.

Look into free public-health clinics, community and rural health centers, or school-based programs.

Finally, you can pay out of pocket. In this case, shop around for quality care at the best price possible. Some doctors, clinics, and hospitals can offer payment plans; unfortunately, many just want you to use a credit card upfront. Ask the billing office to see what options may be available for the balance of your payments.

read and consider them thoughtfully (and have a trusted friend or family member read them as well).

To deem a treatment medically necessary, the insurer will require written notice from your doctor that the treatment is required for your care. Based on how well your doctor documents the need for the treatment or test, along with how the general medical community considers the necessity of it, your insurer will make a subjective decision. Many times you can change an insurance company's decision by asking your doctor's office to contact the insurance company and provide more information about the need for the care. Sometimes the problem is as simple as correcting an incorrect code that was submitted to the insurance company by a billing clerk! What if you do all of that and you still strike out? If you have employer-sponsored health insurance, contact the human resources department at your workplace. The benefits manager there may help you negotiate with your carrier for an out-of-contract benefit. A patient of mine did just that and was able to return to work with a more specialized wheelchair than the standard chair the insurance company was willing to provide.

In addition to your company's human resources department, also enlist the help of a social worker or case manager from your hospital or physician's office. These individuals can help provide a solid rationale based on medical need for your treatment or device, proving to your carrier that the drug, treatment, or device is not experimental and is absolutely medically necessary.

KNOW HOW HOSPITALS AND CLINICS WORK

As a survivor, you want to stay out of hospitals. That said, from time to time, you may need tests and hospital procedures. During those times, it helps to know the system.

Hospitals and clinics compete with one another. Many of them advertise certain types of care on billboards and television commercials to attract your business. Never assume, however, that just because you saw a service in an ad that it's actually available. Call the hospital and find out what services and resources they can offer, given the health problem you want help with and your insurance. To sort through the marketing and arrive at a confident decision on a hospital or clinic, consider the following:

Branding: One aspect of competition that has emerged among many of the most prominent leaders in the field, such as the Mayo Clinic, the Rehabilitation Institute of Chicago, and Partners Health Care, is the use of their name as a way of "branding" their care. For example, Johns Hopkins Hospital may partner with a hospital in the suburbs that may not have yet established the same level of quality of the main hospital. Therefore, when you are looking into the quality of a program, don't stop with just the name, because the partner may not yet deliver care in a particular area at the same level for which the main program has developed a strong reputation.

Hospital ratings: Several sources of hospital rating systems are available. Your insurance company may maintain a list. Medicare and Medicaid (www.cms.hhs.gov) also provide assistance.

You can also use the commercial Web site HealthGrades.com (www. healthgrades.com). This site creates a ranking of hospitals based on the number of patients who have died (mortality rate) or those who had complications in relation to the number of people expected to have died or had complications during the same period of time. It may not seem to be the best way to determine the quality of a hospital—based on counting the number of people who died—but this is a system that has been long used to measure outcomes in hospitals.

Using this site, you can select your hospital to see how it performs on a variety of specialty-care areas. The highest-rated hospitals receive five stars. The hospitals that receive three-star ratings perform as expected or "average." The one-star rating indicates a hospital that performed more poorly than expected. Also, you should know that researchers do take into account differences in the patients when they report these rankings or assign the stars. This is called "risk adjustment." This is important, because sometimes patients with greater needs go to larger university hospitals and not small community hospitals. In the end, the university hospital may have a higher mortality rate—because patients walk in the door in worse shape than patients who go to other hospitals.

Accreditation: To receive Medicare reimbursement, hospitals must be accredited by the Joint Commission of Accreditation of Healthcare Organizations or by their state's Department of Public Health. So, when a hospital advertises that it is "accredited," don't let it sway your decision. So is every other hospital in your area!

That said, some hospitals can receive specialized accreditation in specific areas such as rehabilitation, pediatrics, and speech pathology. If a hospital has this special accreditation in an area you need treatment, then it stands out from other hospitals that do not.

The Truth About Unequal Care

HEALTH CARE IS not provided equally to all people. First, whether we have insurance, and the restrictions that may carry, definitely affects the type of care we get, how quickly we can receive it, or where we can go for services. Second, there is a lot of research on how things like race/ethnicity, age, and whether you are male or female can impact the care you are able to get. Although there are laws in this country about discrimination, sometimes the fact that you live in an area that does not get as much federal funding, for example, may impact the types of care available.

I am not stereotyping, but alerting you to what really goes on so that you can prevent such neglect in your case. A 2005 study from the University of Maryland reports that minorities were less likely to be treated for cancer than were whites. Also, research shows that women do not receive the same quality of care as men. A Kaiser Family Foundation study in 2004 found that women are more likely to make sure their family members receive care before they take care of themselves. Women are also more likely than men to have difficulties with being able to afford their medications.

A good way to ensure that you are receiving the highest quality of care is to consult the clinical practice guidelines I mentioned earlier. They are objective and will help to ensure your care is meeting the optimal guidelines agreed upon by clinical experts. You can also consult the Web site www.patientinform.org, a site developed by the American Cancer Society, the American Diabetes Association, and the American Heart Association. It offers free access to medical journal articles on cancer, heart disease, and diabetes, with user-friendly explanations of the articles' implications for your health. These groups review hundreds of studies, translate them into plain English, put them in the context of other studies and current practices, and describe how patients and their caregivers can use the knowledge. The site also includes a very good description of what to look for in medical research, and how to assess the quality of a study's design.

Area of specialty: Some hospitals specialize in programs, such as cancer care or cardiac care, for example. These programs are focused on the specific condition; therefore, it is sometimes thought that they can provide high-quality specialty services more efficiently than general hospitals. However, these types of specialties are not "accredited"—they are built on reputation.

KNOW THE LAWS

Laws form the glue that holds that various fragments of the health-care system together. These laws protect your privacy, help you better understand the consequences are of certain diagnostic and treatment options, and ensure that your wishes are adhered to. Know and understand them. They will help you better navigate the system.

Patient Rights and Responsibilities

◈

YOU HAVE SPECIFIC rights as a patient.
They include the right to:

- Privacy
- Access to care
- Read your medical records
- Refuse treatment
- Informed consent
- Understand your bill for the care you actually received

INFORMED CONSENT

Hospitals and physicians will ask you to sign "informed consent" forms. These forms typically cover the following:

- The nature of the decision/procedure
- Any other reasonable alternatives to the proposed procedure. For example, instead of surgery, is there a medication to treat your condition?
- The risks, benefits, and uncertainties related to each alternative
- How well you understand the procedure
- Your willingness for and acceptance of the proposed procedure

This is a lot of information! It is intended to protect you, as well as the physician and hospital. You have the right to read the form and understand what it says before you sign it. The hospital or doctor must explain it to you in a language and a manner that you can understand. Your doctor, hospital, or other provider must explain how a treatment works, its side effects, and alternatives to that treatment. You have a right to know, so always ask. Always get the right form for your specific situation, read it, and ask questions if things are confusing or unclear.

HIPAA and Need for Access to Medical Information

Health-care providers cannot share your information without your knowledge. All doctors now ask you to fill out HIPAA forms (as mentioned earlier, HIPPA is the Insurance Portability and Accountability Act of 1996) almost as soon as you walk in the door. These forms stipulate that some information must be shared for treatment and billing purposes, but also that your information would not be used for marketing purposes. Basically, the intent is to not restrict quality of care, but rather limit access to your personal health information. You can find more information on this law at www.hhs.gov/ocr/hipaa.

HIPAA also requires insurers to cover you if you change from one carrier to another. In the past, if you had a preexisting condition (such as cancer), your employer's insurance company did not have to provide coverage for care related to that condition. This is called "preexisting condition exclusion." Now, the law has changed.

The interactive Web site www.cms.hhs.gov/hipaa is a federally sponsored site that can help you determine your rights and protections under HIPAA. You can also contact the CMS central office at 1-877-267-2323, ext. 61565, for assistance.

Medicare Rights

As with other forms of insurance, you also have the right to complain about your concerns about quality of care if Medicare covers you. On the Medicare Web site (www.medicare.gov), you can obtain phone numbers by state and by type of situation about which you wish to complain. You are allowed to appeal decisions and discuss your Medicare bill or denial of services. Before you go to that level, however, ask your provider to help clarify a billing situation. It may save you time and inconvenience.

ANGIE'S STORY

That's a lot to digest, I know. That said, the information you've absorbed in this chapter will go a long way toward helping improve your health and quality of life. I know it did for Angie, one of Patricia's patients.

Angie is a breast cancer survivor who lives in a rural part of the country with limited access to health-care facilities. When she was first diagnosed, she contacted the only university in the area to arrange for her care. She lived many miles from any other source of care, so she had to rely on this university hospital.

Angie felt that she had to increase her confidence with her choice of care, so she asked friends and neighbors about their experiences with the university hospital. She also joined a local support group, whose members told her what the university hospital was like for initial care and long-term follow-up care during survivorship. Angie also surfed the Internet to find out more about this hospital. Most important, she kept in constant contact with her insurance case manager.

Angie had the support of her church so there, too, she asked about the doctors and the care at the university hospital. Her friends there confirmed the good care that the support group members told her about, but told her to be assertive with her care needs. In other words, they told her to stay on top of her doctor and not to be afraid to call her if she felt at all anxious or concerned about her care.

Pulling in other specialists, Angie used an acupuncturist to help with her feelings of fatigue. She found emotional strength in her church and her religious practices.

Now, two years after her initial diagnosis, Angie has dyed her hair red. At first, the choice was cosmetic. She wanted to cover up the gray induced by her radiation treatments. Now, however, the red is a symbol of her survivorship. Thanks to her doggedness at working the system, Angie is thriving. We hope her story inspires you to become a savvy survivor, too.

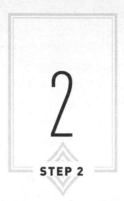

STEP 2

Become a Savvy Survivor

THREE MONTHS INTO my chemotherapy treatment (postradiation), I began to have problems remembering and organizing tasks. People told me to take it easy, slow down, and simplify my life. Co-workers and friends told me they experienced memory lapses, too, even though they had not undergone surgery, radiation, and chemotherapy to treat a brain tumor. Still, I was frustrated.

Despite the fact that a brief test revealed no cognitive deficits and the specialist told me that my brain function was normal for my age, the memory and organizational challenges I faced were not normal *for me*. I wanted answers, so I talked to other survivors with similar challenges, looked up studies about memory and cognitive functioning after chemotherapy, and consulted another specialist at MD Anderson Cancer Center in Houston. She tested my cognitive abilities with more sensitive neuropsychological tests and suggested a number of strategies to help me improve my memory and organization skills at work. She also recommended I take a stimulant medication to help with memory, concentration, and planning.

The medication dramatically improved the situation. After taking it for about six months, however, my blood pressure crept upward. I faced a tough decision. The treatments I received for my brain tumor had already increased my risk for a stroke, and higher blood pressure increased this risk even more. I needed the stimulant medication to perform almost like I did in the past, which is what I was looking for, but taking it could prove disastrous in the long term.

I decided to stop taking the medication. I've since explored other options, including fine-tuning the strategies that the specialist at MD Anderson suggested. I have learned, for example, to respond to e-mails as soon as I read them (so they don't slip my memory). I also write down religiously tasks for the day as well as notes from my conversations with others. I use a calculator rather than figure out simple math in my head.

I tell you this story so you can understand just how important persistence affects health and mental well-being after cancer. I could have given up after that first doctor told me nothing was wrong but, instead, I decided to listen to that inner voice that kept prompting me to explore other options. It worked. I'm a more functional, happier, and healthier survivor as a result.

You must do the same. Whenever you feel that inner voice telling you that a certain symptom or sensation isn't normal—listen! Then, doggedly look for answers. Studies conclusively show that patients who take an active role in their medical care report less physical discomfort, experience less anxiety about their illness, and feel more in control of their illness and more satisfied with their physicians. In this chapter, you'll find everything you need to know to become an expert patient, one who can find and understand quality research and make informed and confident decisions about tests and treatments.

You've already learned how to choose the best physicians in the business. Now, it's time to put them to work for you. The more you know about your condition, symptoms, and possible treatments, the better you will be able to work with your health-care team to get the treatments you need at an affordable price—and improve your health and quality of life as a result.

SAVVY TACTIC #1:
Find and Interpret Information

JOAN, A PITUITARY cancer survivor, returned to work part-time four months after surgery to remove a tumor on her pituitary gland. When she increased her work hours, however, she began experiencing strange symptoms. At times, for seemingly no reason, her heart raced and she couldn't catch her breath. "I just thought my body was not used to this and needed to adjust," she told me. "One day I felt faint. My blood pressure was 170/156 so I rushed to my hospital. They gave me a tablet and an injection to bring down my pressure and sent me home to rest."

After a few weeks, she again returned to work, only to find her racing heartbeat to resurface. Her physician told her that she probably took on too much too soon. "One doctor said I should be better by now; another said everyone heals differently, and just don't rush it. I was told that the tumor was in a place where my hormones are controlled. It is where our powerhouse for our body is; it is off balance, so anything is possible."

She wanted answers, so she did some searching on the Internet. Through the Internet, she found a clinic that specialized in her type of cancer. After battling with her HMO, she eventually got the coverage she needed to go to the clinic, which diagnosed her with an endocrine imbalance. After taking medication to treat this disorder, her symptoms are now under control.

Joan's research (not to mention her persistence with her HMO) paid off. Similar skills can help you as well.

Television, newspapers, and Web sites provide more health information

What You Need to Know About: Virtual Doctors

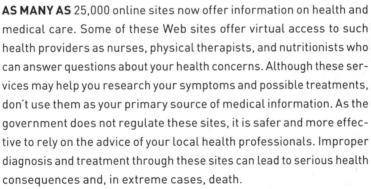

AS MANY AS 25,000 online sites now offer information on health and medical care. Some of these Web sites offer virtual access to such health providers as nurses, physical therapists, and nutritionists who can answer questions about your health concerns. Although these services may help you research your symptoms and possible treatments, don't use them as your primary source of medical information. As the government does not regulate these sites, it is safer and more effective to rely on the advice of your local health professionals. Improper diagnosis and treatment through these sites can lead to serious health consequences and, in extreme cases, death.

On the other hand, more and more doctors are developing their own Web sites to help them stay in touch with their patients. Called "patient-provider portals," these secure Internet-based sites contain a range of software tools and functions. Research suggests that these portals can improve the processes, outcomes, and quality of care. When used in conjunction with face-to-face visits, these sites can help both you and your doctor stay on top of continuous long-term follow-up care by providing you with information and a graphic display of just how well you are responding to a new medication or lifestyle change.

now than ever before. To become a savvy survivor, you must learn how to sift through that information, separating what's accurate and useful from what's false and useless. Pay attention to your knee-jerk reactions, but be aware that your emotions may override your usual common sense! Advertisements for products and services, for example, use attractive marketing hooks to draw you in, triggering an emotional reaction that makes you want the drug or service—right now!—and cause you to look at the information they provide with a less critical eye. I give you these words of advice: don't go there! I've learned this from experience, because, of course, I *have* gone there and gotten swept up by the dramatic claims these advertisers make. At first, you feel an emotional high—you've finally stumbled across the miracle drug or device that will solve all of your problems—that is eventually followed by a dark emotional low when you realize that the drug or device is not the answer you've been waiting for.

The tools you will find in the pages that follow will help you more effectively sort through health information, so that this type of emotional reaction will happen less and less often. Here, you'll find the benefits—and common pitfalls—of different types of health information sources.

The Internet

Perhaps nothing has changed health and health care more than has the Internet. Although the Internet is a valuable resource, you must thoughtfully consider the information you find. This medium offers lots of valuable information at your fingertips at any time of the day or night; however, not all Web sites offer reliable information; also, not all the information you find will apply to your specific situation. Many Web sites, for example, overstate the track record of certain types of alternative remedies and supplements, whereas others understate the value of various treatments. To figure out which sites you can trust, consider the following:

Did a reputable organization or a person create the Web site? In general, information presented on sites created by such national organizations as the National Cancer Institute, is more trustworthy than information from personal Web sites, such as John Brown's Cancer Library. Personal Web sites often offer more opinion than fact.

If it's a personal Web site, can you verify this person has expertise in this area? You can probably trust a site created by a physician or another

Quality Web Sites

THE FOLLOWING WEB sites make a clear distinction between sponsored and editorial content, and used peer-reviewed information written by health professionals.

http://my.web.md
www.nih.gov
www.mayoclinic.com
www.medicinenet.com
www.kidshealth.com
www.medscape.com

professional (although even these sites may be biased toward these doctors' particular views). Be cautious about sites created by those who have struggled with your condition. Again, personal sites often offer opinions and emotional responses to the condition, not unbiased research or facts.

Does a reputable organization, such as a hospital, university, or government organization, sponsor the site? Organizations such as Harvard's School of Public Health, Cedars Sinai Hospital, and the Centers for Disease Control have no ulterior motive; their goal is to provide you with information you need to get better. However, many other organizations, such as drug companies, create some Web sites for the main purpose of selling or marketing a product.

When the site makes a claim about a treatment or drug, does it also provide information about who originally made the claim, why, and when? For example, if a site claims that a new drug can shrink a tumor; does it offer published studies to back up the statement or is it just someone's story of how it works? Make sure the published article comes from a reliable source. (You'll learn later in this chapter how to judge the accuracy of medical studies.)

Weigh the information you find on the site against information you receive from other trusted sources, including your doctor. Although a Web site may offer accurate information about various approaches

Web Site Quality Assessment

TO FIGURE OUT which sites you can trust, use this checklist.

1. Look at the Web site address—does the address make sense for the type of information presented?	Yes	No
2. Is it a personal Web site?	Yes	No
3. If so, can you find out more about this person to verify he or she has expertise in this area?	Yes	No
4. Is the site sponsored by a reputable organization?	Yes	No
5. Are claims referenced?	Yes	No
6. Do the links work?	Yes	No
7. Do other major organizations link to this site?	Yes	No
8. Is there a date on the site to show when it was posted?	Yes	No

All of these answers should be Yes except for question number 2, which should be No.

to the challenges you might face, working with your doctor can help you figure out whether those treatments will work for your specific situation. To make the best use of the Internet, use the Web Site Quality Assessment.

Libraries

Your librarian can help you find books, videos, and articles that relate to your problem. Most libraries—even if they don't hold the volume you need—can access what you need from another library through interlibrary loans.

In addition to consulting your local library, visit the patient library or education room at your local hospital. Hospital staff can usually help you more effectively search the Internet as well as provide books, videos, and other handouts on your condition. Large hospitals affiliated with universities often house more information than small ones. Even if you are not a current or past patient of one of these large hospitals, you can probably still access its patient-education room.

Bookstores

At your local bookstore, you'll find many books (such as the one you are reading right now!) about the challenges of cancer and related health issues. Although you will probably find more up-to-date books at these bookstores than at your local library, these books can also become outdated. Check the copyright date, selecting books that were published during the past one to two years. Also, many self-help books describe one individual's experience; what worked for him or her may not work for you. Read such books with a careful eye and talk to your health-care providers about any questions or concerns that arise.

Community or National Advocacy Groups

Advocacy groups, particularly those on a national level, often provide free educational materials. Many of these organizations have a help line you can call. Staff will listen to your questions and concerns, suggest additional information, and refer you to health-care providers, support groups, and activities in your local area. You'll find contact information for many of these organizations in Appendix A.

Your Health-care Team

Your doctor, nurse, or physician's assistant can provide information and handouts about your illness and symptoms. Although these health-care professionals are trained to educate and provide information, they can become very busy and sometimes too busy to provide full answers. The typical doctor's visit lasts just seven to ten minutes. The more you research beforehand, the more effectively you will ask questions—and get answers—during those few precious minutes.

Family and Friends

Your friends and family members can help you gather information, allowing you to focus on your care. Make sure they apply the same high standards to the quality of information they gather as you would if you were doing it yourself. You can also lean on friends and family when you need to make important decisions. Talking with them about the situation can help you feel more in control.

The News Media

You no doubt have encountered plenty of health information in newspapers, magazines, and on the six o'clock news. Although these sources can help keep you on your toes and point you to research that you didn't know about, they can also bombard your with untrustworthy information. When you obtain information from news media, confirm it with your health-care provider and search for medical studies that back it up.

Medical Studies

Of all sources of information about cancer and cancer survivorship, medical studies are generally the most reliable. That said, you can't believe everything you read in a study (and you'll soon find out why.) You'll find two main types of medical studies. The more prevalent of the two, single studies, examine a particular topic. These studies start out with a hypothesis or idea, create an experiment to test that hypothesis, and describe the results based on that experiment. Although results of initial single studies may be exciting, don't bet your house on their results. According to a recent report in the *Journal of the American Medical Association,* 16 percent of initial studies completed on a drug, treatment, or test were contradicted in future studies. Also, when studies that initially showed an intervention was superior or critical were completed again, only 44 percent of those studies reported the same results as the original study.

So what do you do? How do you know whether to trust a study result? For most of your medical research, rely on a second type of study, known as a *review article* or *meta-analysis,* also called a "study of studies." These reviews look at the existing research studies on a topic, weigh the available evidence, and arrive at a conclusion based on that evidence. Typically meta-analyses ask a specific question, such as "What is the effectiveness of pain medication for breast cancer survivors?" or "Are different types of pain medication more effective than others for cancer pain in certain forms of cancer?" From these initial questions, researchers search key databases of scientific studies, such as Medline, the Cochrane Library, and Cancerlit (a source of cancer-related research articles). They often start with thousands of studies. After tossing out poorly designed and biased studies, however, they actually examine only hundreds. For example, one meta-analysis I came across recently looked at 25,000 articles. After separating the wheat from the chaff, however, it actually examined 213 specific studies.

The Cochrane Collaboration, an international nonprofit organization that provides current information about the effects of health care, completes meta-analyses on a regular basis. These reviews can help you see how the research stacks up for different types of remedies and treatments. Whereas a single study might have hidden biases or sloppy methodology, modern reviews—especially a Cochrane review—generally excludes studies with such problems. Unlike some studies, Cochrane reviews generally are written in easy-to-understand language as well. You can find free abstracts of these reviews by visiting the Cochrane Web site (www.cochrane.org).

Cochrane and other types of reviews help to put contradictory single studies in perspective. To rely on medical information, you need repeated studies completed by different research groups, with many patients. When study results are similar from one project to the next, the findings become more and more likely to be true, valid or believable.

You, Too, Can Read Medical Journals

You don't need a medical degree or doctorate to understand scientific research. To prove this point, let's take a look at a hypothetical scenario. Let's say you hear a news report, based on a study in the *New England Journal of Medicine,* which says exercise reduces fatigue in cancer survivors. You want to read more.

First, you need to get a copy of the article. To do so, write down everything you remember from the report, including the name of the journal, the title of the study, the date it was published, the authors' names, and the basic details about the study. Then either go online to the National Library of Medicine's search database (www.pubmed.gov) or head to your local library.

The National Library of Medicine's database (commonly called "Medline" and "Pubmed") indexes roughly 4,800 journals, including only those journals that a team of reviewers determine to provide unique, scientifically worthy, quality research on a consistent basis. If you use the National Library of Medicine's database, enter simple search terms, such as "fatigue," "cancer survivor," or "exercise." If you type in too much information, the database will not be able to track down studies that match your result.

If you type in too little, you'll end up with hundreds of studies to read through—and not enough time to read them all.

When searching a medical database such as Medline, follow these steps:

1. **Determine the topic.**
   What is the topic you wish to learn more about? Write down the question you want to answer in the space provided.

   Write your question here: _____

   _____

2. **Determine your keywords.**
   Based on your question, list three to five specific keywords that describe your topic.

   List your key words here: _____

   _____

   Let's say you are interested in learning about ways to cope with worries related to work. Your keywords might include: "anxiety," "treatment," "cancer," "survival," "work."

   Try typing those words into an Internet search engine or use a thesaurus to find similar words that may be more recognizable in the scientific literature. Consult a medical librarian at your local medical school library or e-mail a cancer organization for help.

3. **Determine your search engine.**
   Possibilities include PubMed (www.pubmed.com), PubMed Consumer Health (http://medlineplus.gov), Cochrane Collaboration Reviews (www.cochrane.org), AHRQ (www.ahrq.gov), and general Internet search engines, such as Yahoo! or Google.

   If you use your local library, ask the librarian for help. Show your librarian your notes and explain what you are looking for. Your librarian will help you track down the study through databases at the library. Try combinations of your keywords to hone your search. For example, first try the phrase "anxiety & cancer" (the "&" symbol will combine the words so you find articles with both anxiety *and* cancer in them.) If you get too many hits, add an additional word, try "anxiety & cancer & work."

4. **Look at the abstracts and/or Web sites.**
   Read through the abstracts to see if they make sense and come close to answering your question. Share these abstracts with your health-care provider for further explanation and clarification of how it may apply to your situation.

5. **Keep notes on your searching steps.**
   Try your search again in a few weeks or months; new things may be published or be posted on Web sites.

Once you have the study in hand, you need to learn how to interpret it. Start with the abstract. It will give you a quick read of the entire article. You'll find the abstract at the very top of the first page; it is usually titled "abstract." To learn how to read an abstract, let's take a look at one I found in the *Journal of Clinical Oncology.* (See Sample Study Abstract on page 44.)

From the abstract, you'll be able to find answers to the following important questions:

Who published it? The sample abstract was published in the *Journal of Clinical Oncology,* a prestigious, peer-reviewed journal. As does the *Journal of Clinical Oncology,* many medical journals hold the articles they publish to a high standard for accuracy, reliability, and usefulness. Before publishing a scientific article, these journals send the proposed article to several reviewers who read the article and offer comments and criticism. These reviewers, often experts on the topic of the article, ensure only quality research gets into the journal. These reviewers can suggest the journal not publish an article or suggest an author revise an article. Only the rare study flies through the review process untouched.

Not all medical journals, however, complete this rigorous process. How can you tell if a journal is high quality? Look at its impact rating. Based on how often studies in the journal are cited in subsequent scientific research, the Institute of Scientific Information (www.isinet.com) each year assigns medical journals a number ranging from 1 to 100. A journal with an impact rating of 100 is one hundred times more likely to be read and cited than one with a rating of 1; the higher the rating, the more prestigious the journal.

Who wrote it? The sample abstract was written by researchers from the faculty of Physical Education, University of Alberta. It even provides their

Sample Study Abstract

Randomized Controlled Trial of Exercise Training in Postmenopausal Breast Cancer Survivors: Cardiopulmonary and Quality of Life Outcomes

J. S. Courneya, J. R. Mackey, G. J. Bell, L. W. Jones, C. J. Field, A. S. Fairey, *Journal of Clinical Oncology* volume 21, issue 9 (May 2003): 1,660–1,668. (Use the volume, issue, year, and page numbers to help you find the article.)

Purpose: To determine the effects of exercise training on cardio-pulmonary function and quality of life (QOL) in postmenopausal breast cancer survivors who had completed surgery, radiotherapy, and/or chemotherapy with or without current hormone therapy use.

Methods: Fifty-three postmenopausal breast cancer survivors were randomly assigned to an exercise (n = 25) or control (n = 28) group. The exercise group trained on cycle ergometers three times per week for 15 weeks at a power output that elicited the ventilatory equivalent for carbon dioxide. The control group did not train. The primary outcomes were changes in peak oxygen consumption and overall QOL from baseline to post intervention. Peak oxygen consumption was assessed by a graded exercise test using gas exchange analysis. Overall QOL was assessed by the Functional Assessment of Cancer Therapy-Breast scale.

Results: Fifty-two participants completed the trial. The exercise group completed 98.4% of the exercise sessions. Baseline values for peak oxygen consumption (p =.254) and overall QOL (p =.286) did not differ between groups. Peak oxygen consumption increased by 0.24 L/min in the exercise group, whereas it decreased by 0.05 L/min in the control group (mean difference, 0.29 L/min; 95% confidence interval [CI], 0.18 to 0.40;p <.001). Overall QOL increased by 9.1 points in the exercise group compared with 0.3 points in the control group (mean difference, 8.8 points; 95% CI, 3.6 to 14.0; p <.001). Pearson correlations indicated that change in peak oxygen consumption correlated with change in overall QOL (r = 0.45; p<.01).

Conclusion: Exercise training had beneficial effects on cardiopulmonary function and QOL in postmenopausal breast cancer survivors.

contact information. This is very helpful, because you can contact the researchers for more information about the study. Many researchers are only glad to help. Most will be flattered that you find their study useful! After all, that is why most of them are doing this work.

To find more information about the study, for example what impact this information might have on your personal situation, contact the lead study author. Generally, you'll find contact information for the lead study author in the lower left-hand corner of the first page or at the very end of the article. If the article does not list an e-mail or snail mail address, you can usually track down the authors by searching the Web sites for the university or institution where they work. Most universities offer a search-able staff database that will yield phone numbers and e-mail addresses for their professors.

What did the authors set out to prove? Using the scientific method that you learned in high school, the study first lays out the background and hypothesis (or question) that the researchers set out to test. For example, in the abstract, the researchers designed a study to answer this question: "What are the effects of weight loss on tumor recurrence in breast cancer?" Some papers call this section the *purpose* or *background* or *objective*.

How did the authors design an experiment to test their hypothesis? After describing the basis for the hypothesis, the article will delve into the *methods*, or how they designed the study. The methods section may seem like a lot of boring details, but you can learn a lot about the quality of the study and whether the results apply to your specific situation if you take your time and explore this section carefully. In the methods section of a study, you can find:

- *The sample size:* Generally, the larger the number of people studied the better.
- *The selection process:* The methods section will list the type of problem, age range, educational background, gender, and ethnicity of study participants, among many other factors. Make sure the study included participants who are like you.
- *The experiment that the researchers designed:* This can give you a good idea about how well the study results apply to real life. Although no study will mimic real life exactly, some come closer than others. For example, if in testing the health benefits of a specific meal plan, researchers fed

participants certain foods in a lab; you might wonder how the results would apply to real life. Would the participants have stuck to the plan if they had to cook the foods themselves at home? Maybe, maybe not.

Take a look at the sample abstract. In the methods section, you'll see that the researchers enrolled twenty-five women in the exercise program and twenty-eight in the *control* (or no-treatment) group, and looked at how each of the groups did in comparison to one another. The article also includes its authors' method for evaluating the information, along with plans for statistical analysis. Don't let the statistics or other formulas scare you off. Other sections of the article will explain what you need to know. You need not understand the numbers!

What did the study find? After the methods section, you'll find a results section, usually chock full of numbers. Again, if it reads like scientific gobbledygook, don't become too concerned. However, it deserves looking at. Sometimes the results section may help you to determine the clinical significance of a study. Many articles depict tables or graphs that describe study results; you might find these useful in understanding the numbers behind a study. They can also help you see just how dramatic (or undramatic) the results really are. For example, many studies focus on a concept known as *statistical significance*. What a statistician considers "significant," however, is much different from what you or I would consider significant. In statistics, the word *significant* does not mean "a lot." It simply means that the test resulted in enough of a change to rule out happenstance. Yet, what was studied may only have had a small effect. For example, a study might find that a certain cancer drug resulted in a "statistically significant" improvement in longevity compared to a placebo, yet the improvement may only have been a few days or weeks longer, which certainly isn't a lot.

What did the researchers conclude based on those results? After the results section, you'll find the discussion and conclusion. These are the pearls of the article. If the study has seemed like Greek to you until now, this section will help. In the discussion, the study authors explain the results of their study. In the sample abstract, the discussion explains that exercise training improved the cardiopulmonary function and quality of life in postmenopausal breast cancer survivors.

Read the discussion and conclusion sections carefully. This section contains information on the study's limitations, aspects about the study design that limit its application. For example, in this section, the authors might explain that their sample (or group of people studied) did not contain any African-Americans, so the study results might not apply to this population of people. In this case, the authors might suggest future research on that population.

After reading the abstract and getting a general idea of what the study found, you're ready to read the full article. The sections of the paper follow the same outline as the abstract, except with much more detail. Use the descriptions of each section of the abstract to guide you as you read the entire article. Again, don't worry if you don't understand all of the language. Pose any remaining questions about the article to your doctor. Take a copy of the article with you to your appointment. Specifically, ask your physician how the results might apply to your situation and whether you could benefit from what the study described.

If your doctor does not agree with the recommendations presented in a particular article, ask why and continue to ask why until you feel satisfied with his or her answers. If, after hearing your doctor out, you feel strongly that the study outlines a treatment that you wish to pursue—regardless of your doctor's opinion—get a second opinion, from another doctor. You can physically visit another doctor within that specialty or contact an academic medical center that handles this type of health problem. Such centers generally take a team approach to your problem with the assumption that your problem may be influenced by or affect many aspects of your life. In one of these centers, one physician will examine your medical health and another will examine your behavioral and psychological health. You may also see nurses, nutritionists, experts in complementary health care, and physical therapists, depending on your symptoms. Staff in these centers stay on top of the new research in many areas related to your specific problem.

SAVVY TACTIC #2:
Make Informed Decisions about Your Care

AFTER MY YEAR-LONG chemotherapy ended, I experienced variations in my mood. I felt okay some days and other days I felt pretty bad. I mentioned the problem to my neuro-oncologist, who explained that the chemotherapy I had undergone probably had altered my brain chemistry, lowering levels of a brain chemical called *serotonin* that promotes feelings of calm and balanced mood. He recommended a low-dose antidepressant to elevate my serotonin levels. A few months after I starting taking the drug, I began

What Is a Quality Study?

ASK YOURSELF THE following questions, developed by researchers from the Research Triangle (a prestigious research institute in North Carolina) when "grading" an article for medical consideration.

WHAT IS A QUALITY STUDY?	
TYPES OF INFORMATION THAT MAY BIAS THE SCIENCE REPORTED IN INDIVIDUAL ARTICLES	
AREA OF CONCERN	POTENTIAL PROBLEM
Who did the study include? Who did it exclude?	If you are a black female older than age 50 but the study only included white males age 25 years old and younger, the results may not apply to you.
How many people did the study include?	A study of just a few people is usually not as reliable as a study or a few hundred or few thousand people. Look in the methods section to find out why researchers used the number of participants.
Who dropped out of the study?	If all of the unhealthy people dropped out, the results will look artificially good because only healthy people remained.
What is the statistical appropriateness of the methodology?	Read the methods section to find out why the researchers used a particular statistical technique or method of dealing with the data analysis. Make sure they reference other research articles to support the method used in this article.
What did the study find and why does it work?	The result should make sense. For example, if an article found that exercise helps improve quality of life, the article should explain why.

gaining weight, a common side effect of this particular medication. I was feeling good, so I stopped taking the antidepressant and my weight stabilized. After about three months without the medicine, however, I began feeling pretty low. I resumed the prescription, but cut the dose in half. In a notebook, I graphed my mood, appetite, and weight. After a few weeks, my notes revealed that the reduced dose solved my problem. I felt better and had not gained any weight.

You, no doubt, have already faced similar decisions during your survivorship journey. As you will discover, you will often have many options, some better than others and many equally effective. Finding the best treatment is not as simple as some people think. In most cases there is no right or wrong way to go.

You can, however, arrive at a confident decision. The following problem-solving technique has been used in businesses and health-care settings for effective decision making with great success. Research shows that this technique can help cancer survivors become more effective decision makers, consequently reducing the depression and anxiety that often accompanies indecision.

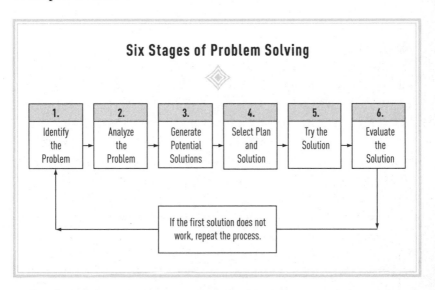

The technique will help you to organize your thoughts and actions, identify the actual problem and solve it. You will follow this process:

- Identify the problem.
- Gather information.

- Develop plans to solve the problem.
- Pick a plan to try.
- Implement your plan.
- Determine whether your plan worked.

To see how you might use this process, let's take a look at how Karen, a patient who was in one of my cancer survivor groups, followed this decision-making process. Several months after her final chemotherapy treatment, Karen returned to work. She experienced ongoing pain, even though many of her other postchemotherapy symptoms had subsided. Karen woke often during the night. Tossing and turning had become a regular occurrence. She felt bone tired most of the day, was gaining weight, felt sad, and had little interest in painting, her favorite hobby. She thought that her major problem was that her pain was disrupting her sleep at night, making her tired during the day. She was not sure for certain, so she used the decision-making process along with her doctor's thoughts to understand what may be happening with her.

Identify the problem. Karen's doctor suggested that depression was probably increasing her pain and setting off the cascade of problems and prescribed an antidepressant. She tells her that medication will not only lift her mood, but also can help reduce the pain, improve sleep, and boost her energy levels. Karen listens, however, she doesn't agree that it's depression and doesn't think the antidepressant will solve her problem. She tells her doctor that her pain is all that she can think of and wonders if the chemotherapy did not completely work, despite what her doctors have told her. Her doctor reassures her, suggesting that she talk to a counselor, because her reactions are not unexpected given all she has been through. She tells her that research has shown that counseling along with an antidepressant is the best treatment for depression.

Gather information. Karen goes online and looks up Web sites and articles about her cancer and pain but also depression and various treatments. She learns that weight gain, sleeplessness, and her lack of interest in painting are all common symptoms of depression. She suspects her fears of cancer are part of her emotional distress. She also found studies where residual pain was made worse by a number of possibilities related to the surgery she had, as well as the pathology of the tumor. She finds information on the treatment of depression that confirms the doctor's advice. Karen now firmly believes that while depression maybe making things worse, she needs to confirm for herself that things are okay inside her body regarding the tumor and surgery as well as looking into medication for depression.

Develop plans to solve the problem. Karen visits her doctor again and discusses various options. Her doctor suggests a repeat MRI, and a follow-up visit with the surgeon along with the antidepressant. She also gives her the phone number to the hospital's mental health clinic to help her find a counselor because the fear of recurrence is getting to her. Karen later learns that insurance will only cover ten sessions of counseling and that her co-pay would be $20 per session. The clinic suggests that she may be able to see a counselor trainee at the local university who is able to see patients without cost.

Pick a plan to try. After considering all of her options, Karen decides to try the antidepressant and not the counseling right away. She decides to wait and see if the antidepressant will work. She also scheduled a visit for follow up with her surgeon.

Implement your plan. Karen fills the prescription, starts the medication, and sees the surgeon with the results of her recent tests.

Determine whether your plan worked. There is no clear evidence of tumor regrowth or major new scar tissue that could clearly account for the persistent pain. Karen feels reassured, and after trying the medication for a month, she notices some improvement.

As you can see, Karen's first go-round with the decision-making process helped, but she's not done yet. Although she's made some improvement, Karen has not completely solved her problem, so she persists, going through the steps again.

Identify the problem. Karen thinks some type of pain management counseling will help with her pain and mood because she still is experiencing pain, which triggers her fear of recurrence. She does not want to take a higher dose of the antidepressant because she really wants to learn how to manage her pain and fear with other approaches. She would like to talk to someone to help her learn pain management approaches, get on with her life, and not always worry about cancer recurrence.

Gather information. Karen visits her doctor again to check whether levels of the medication are at the correct dosage, and to tell her about the pain management option and counseling regarding the fears. Her doctor knows of a pain program in the university medical center that offers counseling and pain management at a sliding fee scale for services not covered by insurance and gives her the phone number to call.

Develop plans to solve the problem. Karen calls the pain program and works out a payment plan for the initial evaluation to see whether the approaches they offer can help her.

Pick a plan to try. Karen decides to go to the pain program for an evaluation.

Implement your plan. She goes for the evaluation. She continues taking her medication and starts seeing a counselor.

Determine whether your plan worked. Within about a month Karen is managing her pain better, sleeping better, feeling more energetic during the day and less fearful. She reports that she feels happier overall. She begins to paint again and realizes that she can paint her story into her work.

As this example illustrates, Karen's persistence paid off. It will for you as well. Use this technique whenever you have decisions to make about your health (or in life in general). It's time you try this process. Use the worksheet on page 53 to help.

Practice Solving a Problem

Let's use the steps you just learned to address a problem that you have. Use the questions below to guide you in this process.

PROBLEM SOLVING WORKSHEET

Identify the problem. *Define it in more detail.*

_____

_____

_____

_____

_____

_____

Gather information. *What seems to be exacerbating and maintaining the problem?*

_____

_____

_____

_____

_____

_____

Develop plans to solve the problem. *The potential plans should be directly related to what you came up with as the factors influencing the problem.*

_____

_____

_____

_____

_____

Pick a plan to try. *Choose something you think will work and is the most likely plan to be attempted.*

_____

_____

_____

_____

_____

_____

Implement your plan. *Just do it. Think of all the barriers to making the plan happen and work through them.*

_____

_____

_____

_____

_____

_____

Determine whether your plan worked. *Choose some way to monitor the outcome. Make sure you follow up. If doesn't work, start again at step 1. Know that this is all part of the process. The first plan you try may not be the one that works. You need to keep trying until the problem is solved.*

_____

_____

_____

_____

_____

_____

Additional Problem-Solving Advice

Whenever I have a tough problem to solve, I like to go through the process using a notebook. It helps me organize my thinking about the problem and gives me an opportunity to generate some realistic potential solutions. I first list the problem. I try to define it as specifically as possible. Then I try to figure out what is influencing it. At this point, I do a little research, using Medline and/or the Internet. I talk to others—my wife, friends, relatives, co-workers, and doctors—to see what solutions might be helpful. Back in my notebook, I generate a list of options with notes about pros and cons. When that list is completed, I choose the option that makes the most sense and often is the easiest to implement. I try it and see if it works. If not, I go back to some other solution on my list and try that one. I don't give up until something works.

I, of course, do not follow this process with every decision I need to make. If I did, I'd never get anything done! I use it only for those mysterious, persistent symptoms or problems. Not only does it help generate a number of potential solutions, it helps me stay in control of my survivorship. I feel better when I know I'm in control!

For best results when making any decision, follow these pointers:

Consider all sources of information. Surf the Internet, talk to friends and other cancer survivors, read medical studies, and, above all else, consult your doctor. Your physician has been studying your condition for years. Make the most of your physician's knowledge!

Communicate assertively. Whether you are seeking advice from your doctor, gathering information from your insurance company, or checking prices on various therapies, ask for what you need—and keep asking until you get an answer.

Trust your instincts. If a problem or solution does not feel right to you, it probably isn't right.

Negotiate for what you need. Don't rule out potential solutions because they seem too expensive or complicated. You never know whether someone is willing to offer you a reduced rate (or even work pro bono) unless you ask. To improve your negotiation outcome, search for a win-win solution.

SAVVY TACTIC #3:
Use Complementary and Alternative Medicine (CAM) Wisely

A YEAR AFTER chemotherapy, I began feeling fatigued again. I thought that maybe my tumor was coming back. This, fortunately, was not the case. Since I had used acupuncture after my radiation to help me with fatigue, I decided to give it another shot.

My doctor didn't think it is worthwhile and told me I was wasting my money.

Yet, each time the acupuncturist treated me, I felt stronger and more alert, relaxed, and more energetic. That's all that mattered. Even if the energy boosting affect was all in my head—what doctors often refer to as "the placebo effect"—I didn't care. As long as I continued to feel better, I decided to keep getting treated. I carefully monitored how I felt after each treatment and through my treatments over time, logging my energy levels on a graph in a journal. If the effect wore off or I was at a plateau that was acceptable to me (that is, my energy was up and I felt okay), I planned to discontinue the treatments. This self-monitoring approach was very help-ful. I stopped treatment after I noticed an improvement in energy for a few weeks in a row. This required about six treatments. I did not go on for as long as the provider thought I should. This was not because I thought that it wouldn't help. I conducted my own cost/benefit audit. I thought that the benefits I felt in terms of increased energy were achieved and incre-mental improvement was not worth the time or money. While this can be dangerous with certain treatments, often times for symptom-management approaches, once things seem under control more of the same may not be warranted—especially if you are doing something in addition to the treatment offered to help manage the symptom. I also began to increase my physical activity.

Acupuncture is one of many complementary and alternative medicine (CAM) techniques that can help cancer survivors to improve their physi-cal, emotional, and spiritual well-being. Such therapies can be especially helpful when conventional medicine is not effective, is not available, is too expensive, or poses too many unfavorable side effects.

You use complementary medicine *in conjunction with* more traditional forms of medicine. For example, you might try massage therapy in addition to a prescribed medicine to reduce anxiety. You use alternative medicine *instead of* traditional medicine. For example, I tried acupuncture rather than taking the stimulant suggested as an option to enhance my energy. What defines the treatment as alternative or complementary is how you use it: *along with* traditional medicine or *instead of* traditional medicine.

Although people have turned to CAM approaches for thousands of years, their widespread use in the United States remains a relatively new option for many. These approaches have gradually emerged over the past two decades in Western countries as tools we patients can use to help us. Because conventional Western medical research is only now seriously examining the practice, its usefulness, and the effects of these techniques, little hard modern scientific research exists to definitely say how well these remedies work or how safe they are. The National Institute of Health's National Center for Complementary and Alternative Medicine has been working to change that. This government-run center offers grants to research institu-tions to study these types of medicine. As a result, hundreds of studies on acupuncture, homeopathy, massage, and other types of CAM have been conducted in the past few years.

To learn more about alternative and complementary therapies, go to the National Institute of Health's free Web site (http://nccam.nih.gov). Here you'll find tips for choosing various types of CAM practitioners, articles that summarize the latest research on various types of CAM techniques, and advisories about specific remedies that may be dangerous. Deeper into that site (search for "clinical trials" in their search field), you'll find a list of ongoing NIH funded research and clinical trials, many of which are actively recruiting participants. The site lists includes a description of the study, the name of the principal investigator conducting the study, and eligibility requirements.

To find a CAM provider, go to www.healthy.net. You'll also find useful information at www.jr2.ox.ac.uk/bandolier/booth/booths/altmed.html, the Web site for *Bandolier,* a journal that examines health-care issues. This site provides current research on complementary and alternative therapies, summarizing the studies in an easy to read manner.

After reviewing these reputable sites, you'll see that the most recent research shows that some CAM remedies can be helpful, especially when combined with conventional treatment. In a study of cancer patients, CAM was found most effective at relieving the side effects of cancer treatment, such as pain, fatigue, nausea, and anxiety. Just fewer than 80 percent of survivors indicated that a combined approach that blended CAM with conventional medicine resulted in better symptom relief than either approach did alone. Because of this, I suggest you consider complementary therapies in conjunction with your mainstream medical care. Also, monitor your results closely. Keep a journal of your symptoms and give whatever technique you try an adequate trial. Above all else, discuss whatever technique you wish to try with your physician. Unfortunately, fewer than 30 percent of patients discuss CAM techniques with their physicians.

In addition to offering information about various types of CAM, your physician can help ensure that the CAM you try does not negatively interact with whatever conventional treatments you are using. This is particularly important if you are taking an herbal supplement or are following a special diet, as these may interact, positively or negatively, with any conventional treatment. For example, a commonly used herb, St. John's Wort, can reduce the therapeutic effects of chemotherapy and could lead to serious consequences.

Although more and more doctors are learning about these approaches, many do not stay abreast of the latest CAM research and some refuse to consider these approaches, for fears of liability or concerns if something goes wrong. If you are interested in trying CAM, but your physician will not discuss the matter with you, you may need to find a doctor who will.

Sometimes a consultation at a medical center with someone who is an expert in this area is helpful. Before searching your provider directory, however, try the following step-by-step strategy for collaborating with your physician about CAM.

1. Identify the most significant symptom you'd like to resolve. Even if you have many symptoms, filter them down to the one or two that bothers you most. For example, if headaches debilitate you more than anything else, start there. Talk to your doctor about this symptom, what in your current treatment regimen or environment might be contributing to it, and what in the world of CAM might help.

2. Keep a symptom diary. In a notebook or PDA, or on a computer, keep track of the time, date, and circumstances of your symptoms. Use a scale of 0 to 10 to indicate the severity of that symptom (consult the Sample Symptom Diary, page 59, for guidance), with 0 meaning you don't notice the symptom at all and 10 meaning it's so severe you cannot function normally.

3. Write everything down. In your symptom diary, write down decisions you and your doctor make together. Also, jot down notes about your sessions with your doctor. Both you and your doctor may find these notes useful later when considering other treatments.

4. Discuss your preferences and expectations with your doctor. Talk to your doctor about your decision to seek CAM therapies. Tell him or her about what you expect from such care. Your doctor may provide some input about additional conventional treatments that may help.

5. Talk to your doctor about safety and efficacy. Your doctor will probably want to help you monitor your health and overall well-being as you pursue your CAM therapy. Ask your doctor how CAM might affect other therapies and medications.

6. Schedule a follow-up visit (or telephone call) to review your treatment plan. Stay in touch with your medical doctor. Either during a quick phone call, in a follow-up with the nurse in the office, mailed written note, or personal follow-up visit, let him or her know your CAM treatment plan.

7. Check in again to review your results. After about four to eight weeks, visit your doctor and go over your experience. Bring your symptom diary to this visit to help jog your memory. At this time, you and your medical doctor can work together to evaluate the

Sample Symptom Diary

USE THE FOLLOWING chart to track your symptoms to see whether a particular treatment is working. For example, on this 0 to 10 scale, you would give no headache pain a 0 and the worst headache pain imaginable a 10. Each time you rate your pain, jot down the time of day and date, and any comments that come to mind. For example, if you didn't sleep well the night before, jot it down. It might explain your symptom. Share your symptom notes with your physician before you start a CAM therapy. Continue using it as you try the approach you decide to use; it will give you objective evidence to gauge the effectiveness of the intervention.

(Note: you can use this form to track any type of symptom or health behavior you want to change, such as exercise, relaxation, weight loss, relationship stress, job stress, or nutrition.)

SAMPLE SYMPTOM DIARY										
SYMPTOM RATING: 0 (no symptom) to 10 (worst imaginable)										
0	1	2	3	4	5	6	7	8	9	10

DATE AND TIME	SYMPTOM EPISODES AND RATINGS

effectiveness of the therapy you tried. If, after this visit, you determine the therapy is not helping, try something else. Don't stick with a therapy that doesn't work!

SAVVY TACTIC # 4:
Find a Patient Navigator

RESEARCHING YOUR SYMPTOMS and communicating with your physician about all your experiences can become tiring, and, as a survivor, energy may already be in short supply. To stay on track, you often can use the help of a *patient navigator*. Although this word sounds as if a legal or medical background is necessary, your patient navigator can be a friend or family member. To some, this function may already be familiar as the term *advocate*—simply meaning someone whom you trust to assist you with regard to research, footwork, and/or communications. My navigator is my wife, Shelley.

Several people can help you negotiate or move through the health-care system, including family members, friends, social workers, case managers, and discharge planners. Such people can help you find a range of services, talk to your insurance company, and/or manage the costs of your care. Most hospitals employ someone on staff who may be able to help you with such matters. These individuals help cancer survivors and others with chronic diseases access care when you need it. These "official" patient navigators ensure that you do not "fall between the cracks," miss important treatments, or leave the health-care system entirely. Consult the American Cancer Society for help in finding a patient navigator (see Appendix A for contact information).

Not only does Shelley, my patient navigator, provide support, she has kept me on top of follow-up medical care. When I was diagnosed with sleep apnea about a year after being diagnosed with cancer, I was prescribed a CPAP (continuous positive airway pressure) unit to wear while sleeping. The mask I needed to wear while I slept was cumbersome and uncomfortable, and after a few attempts to work with it I stopped using it.

Shelley kept on me to go see another sleep specialist. So after sleeping without the unit for about eight months, I finally went to see another sleep expert. I hesitated because I simply did not want to go to another doctor for awhile. As it turned out, the dose of airflow the other sleep lab recommended was excessively high (twice as forceful as it needed to be), making for a very uncomfortable situation. The second sleep expert recommended a major reduction in the airflow setting and a more modern less cumbersome mask. Now I can tolerate the device.

Thanks to the second sleep expert and to Shelley for prompting me, I no longer snore. More important, I feel more energetic during the day and, because I no longer stop breathing at night, I'm not taxing my heart. Shelley's assistance has helped me to both survive (I'll live longer) and thrive (I feel better). Choosing her as my patient navigator was quite possibly the savviest decision I have ever made—short of marrying her!

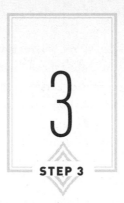

3

STEP 3

Communicate More Effectively

I **ONCE INTERVIEWED** a cancer survivor named Jane. She had been feeling very down, so her doctor prescribed antidepressants to help lift her mood. She had been taking them for three months with no results. She had actually seen her doctor a few times during this time span, but whenever he asked her how things were going, Jane answered, "I'm fine."

I asked her, "Why didn't you tell your doctor that the antidepressants aren't working?"

She replied, "My doctor told me it would take a whilefor it to work."

Something didn't sound quite right to me, so I confirmed some suspicions and looked up information about the drug Jane's doctor had prescribed. It turned out that by "a while," Jane's doctor meant roughly three weeks. Had Jane spoken up and told her doctor that she still felt depressed; her doctor would probably have prescribed a different antidepressant or changed the dosage!

Jane's story illustrates just how much your communication skills can affect your interactions with your physicians and your resulting treatment. Unfortunately, all too often, the typical doctor-patient relationship relies on fractured communication at best. In a study of 1,000 doctor-patient interactions published in the *Journal of the American Medical Association*, patients felt that doctors did not give them enough information to make an informed treatment decision in 91 percent of the cases. In another study, one in four patients said they did not mention their biggest concerns because their doctor didn't ask. Yet another study determined that 80 percent of physicians feel patients participate in decisions, whereas only 30 percent of patients feel this is the case. Finally, research shows that providers underestimate the distress caused by side effects of cancer treatments.

The good news in all of this: you don't have to become one of the statistics that I just mentioned. By learning some simple communication tactics, you can get the information you need to make informed treatment decisions, becoming one of the 75 percent of survivors who feel free to mention their concerns with their doctors and one of the 70 percent of patients who feel they participate in their treatment decisions. Effective communication skills will improve your care in the following ways:

1. **Good follow-through:** When you understand why a treatment is important or how to execute it, you will more likely follow your doctor's instructions. For example, you will try a medication for a sufficient time for it to work rather than stop because of side effects. You'll make follow-up visits, knowing how important it is to get periodic blood tests for glucose you are trying to work so hard on reducing.

2. **Correct medicines and dosages:** Although your doctor often makes an educated decision about what type, brand, and dosage of a medicine you need, given your problem, not all medicines work similarly in all people. So following up and letting him or her know what you are experiencing with a medication will help him or her to fine-tune the dosage and type to your individual situation, reducing side effects and your symptoms. You may, of course, have to try a few different types and dosages of medication before you find one that works for your symptom. If you don't tell your doctor how you feel and how your medicines are working—or not working—you may end up like Jane, taking medicine that doesn't work and suffering unnecessarily with symptoms that could have been solved months ago.

3. **Referrals to specialists:** In these days of managed care, often times you must ask your primary doctor for a referral to a specialist. If you're afraid to speak up, you'll never get the important referral you need to diagnose and treat a specific problem that crops up and may require a specialist's care.

4. **Avoiding health problems due to drug interactions:** Most cancer survivors see different physicians to treat a number of different symptoms. When you speak up and tell each of your physicians about

all of the medications you are taking or the different approaches you are using to solve a problem, you prevent your doctors from accidentally prescribing drugs that reduce the effectiveness of other drugs you are taking or, even worse, cause side effects, such as headaches or fatigue.

Good communication is important for all patients and their doctors, but particularly important for cancer survivors. As a whole, we survivors generally are taking more medications, are seeing more physicians, and have more symptoms that we want to resolve than does the general population. We also need to stay as healthy as we can so we don't wind up with some other illness, such as heart disease or diabetes. To get the best care possible, we survivors need clear and regular communication with our health-care providers to make the best decisions about addressing new problems, monitoring our health, and changing course if necessary. To figure out what the latest research means for us and make informed decisions, we must communicate with our providers and staff in a constructive way.

The skills you will learn here will also help you to better communicate your needs outside of the doctor's office. Having problems with an insurance company, your boss, or a friend? The strategies in this chapter will probably help. The more you assertively—but not angrily—voice your needs and explain your side of a story, the more people will understand you and your situation.

> ### Survivor Stat
>
> ACCORDING TO one survey, cancer survivors who felt comfortable communicating with their health-care providers reported greater satisfaction with their care, a stronger sense of confidence in their abilities to cope with cancer, and better quality of life than patients who were less positive about their communication skills.

GOOD DOCTORS MAKE IT EASY

ACCORDING TO RESEARCH, doctors who do the following during visits tend to make patients feel more comfortable and satisfied with their care, making it easier for patients to speak up:

- Showing a real interest in you as an individual
- Asking about your reasons for coming in and seeking help

- Asking what you think is wrong or what might be causing the symptoms
- Asking how you feel about the situation and its impact on your daily life, mood, and personal relationships

If your doctor follows this process at every visit, your job as an assertive patient will be much easier! Because your doctor asks questions, you'll more easily find the courage to talk about your symptoms, find out information that you need, and as a result, follow through on your doctor's recommendations. To determine whether your doctor enables good communication, consider the following questions:

1. Does my doctor spend enough time listening to my concerns?
2. Does my doctor provide enough information in language I can understand about my symptoms, what might be contributing to them, and what might improve them?
3. Does my doctor provide enough information about my prognosis or what I can expect down the line?
4. Does my doctor share enough information with me about my treatment?
5. Does my doctor ask me if I have any problems with my mood or my relationships or other emotional or personal matters of this type?
6. Does my doctor discuss ways for me to improve my level of social support?

If you are working with one of the best doctors in the business, you might have answered yes to every single question. Of course, not all visits will cover all these things nor do they have to but, over the long run, your doctor should hit all six areas periodically.

What if your doctor falls short? Is it time to find a new doctor? Not necessarily. Although great doctors help to enable great doctor-and-patient communication, that's only part of the communication equation. The other part? You. Throughout this chapter, you will find numerous strategies that will help you to make your doctor's visits

Survivor Stat

IF FERTILITY is a concern, speak up! A study of 657 young cancer survivors found that 72 percent of women discussed fertility concerns with their doctors, and 51 percent felt their concerns were addressed adequately.

as productive as possible. As an added bonus, most of these strategies will work in all areas of your life. Feeling nervous about asking your boss for an accommodation at work? Do you need to find a way to coax a family member or friend into lending you more support? Do you want to tell your friends to stop avoiding conversations about cancer?

USE THE POWER OF THE PEN

A CANCER SURVIVOR I know named Dan told me that he rarely remembered to tell his doctor everything that was on his mind. He went to each visit with the best of intentions yet, during his visit, he would become engrossed in a conversation about one issue and then forget to address another. During his drive home, Dan often thought of questions that he should have asked or symptoms that he wished he had mentioned. Dan was assertive and took his health seriously, so he often scheduled follow-up appointments with his doctor to get all of his questions answered. Still, the issue was becoming frustrating.

I suggested he write down his symptoms and questions beforehand. I mentioned a study that determined patients communicated their symptoms more effectively when their doctors gave them a set of questions to answer before the visit. The questions asked the patients about their symptoms, side effects, and other medical and nonmedical concerns. The doctor was able to review the completed form before seeing the patient, giving him or her a chance to get an idea of some of the patient's concerns.

I suggested that Dan create his own set of questions, one that he could fill out at home and then hand to the receptionist or intake nurse when he got to the doctor's office. Once he began doing so, he was able to get most of his questions answered in just one visit. Even more important, his doctor was so impressed that he began handing a similar form out to other patients to fill out before their visits!

You can do the same. On page 68, you'll find the form, Questions to Ask My Doctor. Photocopy it and use it to jog your memory before each doctor's visit. Take it with you to your visits to help both you and your doctor address all of your questions and concerns.

Don't feel as if you are being pushy. Many patients do this—in fact, many doctors encourage them to do so. Your doctor is probably used to it. To further help you remember everything you want to say, consult the

Questions to Ask My Doctor

THIS FORM WILL help you remember to get all your questions /concerns covered. Don't forget that some of your questions can be answered by the nurse(s) in the office as well. Photocopy this form. Before each visit, write down the questions in each area that are relevant.

Date:
Doctor:

Topic Areas

1. Symptoms

_____
_____
_____
_____
_____

2. Follow-up, future tests, and treatment

_____
_____
_____
_____
_____

3. Prognosis, future treatment

_____
_____
_____
_____
_____

4. Current test results

_____
_____
_____
_____
_____

5. Information

_____
_____
_____
_____
_____

6. Medication

_____
_____
_____
_____
_____

7. Emotional factors

_____
_____
_____
_____
_____

8. Social factors—relationships/support/work/family

_____
_____
_____
_____
_____

9. Family risk

_____
_____
_____
_____

10. Others

_____
_____
_____
_____
_____

following list of typical concerns of cancer survivors. This list of topics is actually based on what other cancer survivors have focused on in their lists, so it probably covers most of the things that you might ever wish to bring up (but of course not everything).

Symptoms:
I now have this persistent back pain for two weeks.
Does the change in hormonal treatment affect my hot flashes?

Follow-up, future tests, and treatment:
When does follow-up for my cancer finish?
Do I need additional chemotherapy?
When will I know whether treatment for the problem has worked?
How do I know the treatment for the cancer has really worked?

Prognosis:
What are my chances of (my problem's) recurrence?
What can I expect in terms of my progress?
Why can disease flare up after tumor removal?

Test results:
Can I actually see my scans?
Can you go over my test results with me? I am confused.
Are you sure they are correct?

Information:
Can you tell me some useful sources of information on the
    problem?
I found this research study; would it apply to me?

Medications:
What are the side effects of the medication you have prescribed
    for me?
How long do I need to take this medication?

Emotional factors:
Are anxiety/panic attacks common in cancer survivors?
I worry about the cancer returning—is that normal?
What can I do when I get down?

Social factors:
Can I now take a job abroad for two years?
Can I take long trips when I don't feel 100 percent?
How do I find help for the stress that comes up with my
spouse now?

Family risk:
Does this cancer run in families?
What are the chances my kids will get this?

GET INSIDE YOUR HEAD

KNOWING YOU CAN and should speak up is one thing, doing it is another. For example, I know a cancer survivor named Sue whom I met a long time ago during a stress management training program I ran. Just a few months ago she relayed a story to me that I would like to share with you.

She said that she had been feeling pretty anxious and her doctor thought she could benefit from a different medication. She told me that she was prescribed the medication at a dose that she felt was contributing to her weight gain, and wanted the dose lowered. Her doctor wanted her to try another antidepressant (common practice—if one does not work, another might) that might not have that side effect. Sue, on the other hand, felt the medicine was helping her. She read that often a reduced dose could prevent weight gain and told her doctor that she wanted try this first. He informed her that he knew what he was doing and a new medication would be the way to go. Sue persisted in a very firm tone, eventually working with her doctor to write the prescription for the same medication at a lower dose and following up. Standing her ground wasn't easy, but she did it because she felt strongly about the matter. She knew from past experience that if she didn't speak up—and let the doctor prescribe a different medication—she probably wouldn't take it and then continue to suffer with the symptoms she was trying to get rid of!

Although most doctors do try to work with you as a partner as much as possible, you do need to make your wishes as clear as you can. To speak up, you first must understand why you *don't* speak up. That varies from person to person, but here are some common beliefs patients have for staying silent:

- **"My doctor is always right and should have the last word when it comes to health matters. After all, he went to medical school; I didn't."** This view is still an extremely common one. Studies tell us most patients are more concerned with following doctor's orders—and in pleasing their doctors—than in participating in decisions. Indeed, in a study of 150 women with breast cancer, only 20 percent wanted to play an active role in their care and only 28 percent wanted to make a joint decision. The remaining 52 percent wanted their doctors to just tell them what to do!

  The reality is this: no doctor is right about everything all the time. Without your input, only the rarest of doctors can make the best recommendations for your care. To recommend the best course of action, your doctor needs you to describe your symptoms and the effects of your treatments in detail. So, you simply can't afford to be passive. You have many options. To stay on top on them, you must talk with your doctor candidly about the pros and cons of each option. If you tend to clam up at the doctor's office because of this flawed belief, tell yourself over and over (silently in your head) that this is *your* health. Only you know your body and mind. Your doctor cannot look at you and guess that there is something wrong. If you are suffering from side effects from medications or treatments or you are not feeling like you generally do, you must tell your doctor. You are not being a hypochondriac. You were diagnosed with cancer. The definition of a hypochondriac is someone who does not have a serious illness, although they may *think* they have one.

- **"If I rock the boat, my doctor will send me packing."** A popular episode of the sitcom *Seinfeld* told the story of Elaine, who ended up on a secret blacklist kept by doctors in her area. She had made the mistake of complaining about side effects of a treatment to one doctor and then, suddenly, all of the doctors in New York City were booked up for months when she called. Although the plot of that episode seems silly, it hints at a fear many of us do hold: that rocking the boat will make their doctor put them on the blacklist. In reality, however, this is very unlikely to happen. Doctors don't desert patients. They have an obligation to help you, so if things are not right, tell them. The vast majority of doctors will work with you to make things better or, if necessary, send you to a specialist who can. To overcome this fear, stay focused. Don't let the visit overwhelm you and feel like you just want to get it over with. This is your chance to let your doctor know what is happening with you. Remind yourself of the old saying, "The only dumb question is the one you didn't ask." It's true. When it comes to your health, there are no dumb questions. You have been through a lot and you can ask anything you want. If you get a blank look or a look of disgust, so what? Your health and well-being are at stake.

■ **"My doctor is very busy. Who am I to take up so much of his or her time? Other patients have more important problems than me."** These days, physicians see more patients and have shorter appointments than ever before. They *are* busy, but they always have been. I'd like to let you in on a little secret. Remember all of that time you spent in the waiting room? You waited in the waiting room because other patients needed time. Your doctor isn't going to tell the last few patients to go home at 5:00 PM because people like you took up too much of his or her time. No, your doctor will continue to see patients until the waiting room is empty. So don't worry about those other patients. It's your doctor's job to spend time with you—and with all of his or her other patients. You are not wasting your doctor's time. If your doctor consistently makes you feel as if you are taking up too much of his or her time, and, you have discussed this with him or her, maybe it's time to find another doctor.

Before your next doctor's visit, take a moment to think about what beliefs or thoughts might be holding you back in the doctor's office. Common thoughts that undermine doctor-patient interactions include the following: "I don't want to look dumb." "I don't want to get her mad at me." "I know she is busy and I don't want to take all of her time." "He can't help me anyway." What thoughts run through your mind just before and during your appointment? What assumptions do you make about your doctor's beliefs, mood, and schedule? Quite often the thoughts and beliefs that stop most people from speaking up stem from incorrect assumptions. For example, you might assume your doctor is in a bad mood or not interested in your problem, but how can you really know unless you bring up the matter?

Whenever you catch yourself thinking such thoughts, replace them with more empowering thoughts, such as the following: "It's her job to listen to me, so I will tell her about this," or "He can only help me if he knows there's a problem." Before your next doctor's appointment, generate a list of some of the problematic thoughts that tend to cause you to clam up. Next to each thought, generate some substitute thoughts that are more realistic. When you head to the doctor's office, have these in the back of your mind. If a negative thought pops up, replace it with a more empowering one from your list. Although this technique requires some practice, it will soon become second nature to you.

Learning to Deal with Uncertainty

MANY SURVIVORS WANT to know whether their cancer will recur, about long-term side effects of their treatments, whether other non-cancer-related health problems might crop up, and how long they really have to live. Don't get too frustrated with your doctor if he or she doesn't give you a clear answer to such questions. It's not that your doctor is trying to avoid your questions. The truth is, there is no clear-cut answer.

Your doctor can of course, based on statistics, give you ballpark guesses as to your odds of survival. But these are only guesses, and they don't get at what's really eating at you: fear.

Life after cancer is ambiguous. This is frustrating at times, of course, but the most successful survivors learn to live with this ambiguity and get on with things. Some seek comfort in religion or spirituality. Some just keep on going with the support of others and their own inner strength. Of course you can do both.

I wish I could answer such questions to eliminate the uncertainty you might feel. Heck, I wish I could put an end to the ambiguity I feel! Alas, this is a battle we must all fight in our own, individual way. To help put ambiguity aside and start living your life again—as you did before cancer—I suggest you change your focus. Instead of looking for a hard number on the number of months or years you have left, focus on how you can maximize your chances of living as healthily as possible, making sure that the quality of that life is good as it can be. Therefore instead of asking your doctor, "How long do I have to live," I recommend you ask the following question: "How can I live longer, with a healthier and a more fulfilled life?"

HOLD A DRESS REHEARSAL

JUNE, A BREAST cancer survivor, had some difficulty getting her doctor to pay attention to her concerns about pain. During one visit, June's doctor had been preoccupied. She'd had an office full of patients and it was already 5:30 PM. June wanted her doctor's full attention. She noticed a picture on her doctor's desk of the doctor's daughter playing soccer. June mentioned that her daughter played soccer, too. All of the sudden, June's doctor became more animated. After talking about soccer for a minute, it seemed as if she were listening a little bit better. The short, personal conversation helped break the doctor out of her rote, quick manner. Both June—and her doctor—benefited from the exchange!

Of course, June handled the situation wonderfully, and not all of us think so quickly on our feet. Handling interactions with your doctor (or your boss or anyone else for that matter) assertively and effectively takes some practice.

Decide what symptom or problem you wish to talk about and then write down how you plan to say it. Then practice. Do it either in front of a family member or friend or in front of a mirror. You might feel silly doing this, but the technique will help you get used to the sound of your own voice. It also will help you to overcome the fear of speaking up. Finally, it will help you to memorize what you want to say. Even if fear or anxiety begins to cloud your brain, your practice sessions will help you to get the words out, almost without really trying. It will help you fine-tune what you want to say, so it more easily spills out of your mouth at the doctor's office, and you will be more comfortable.

Now you know how to counter negative thoughts and how to practice what you want to say. So let's do just that. Let's practice how you might handle a hypothetical problem at the doctor's office, one that tends to cause patients to clam up.

Let's say your doctor prescribes a medication for pain, but you do not completely understand why and how you need to take it. You ask your doctor to explain how the medication works and he seems frustrated that he has to repeat himself. He gives you a quarter of the information he gave you earlier and seems to use more medical jargon this time. What do you do? Most patients would respond in one of the following three ways:

A. You try to listen to the new explanation, but don't ask any more questions because you don't want to upset him any more.

B. You find another doctor and tell that doctor how bad your last one was.

C. You listen to the explanation, and then let your doctor know that you do not understand. You ask him more questions until you do understand.

You, of course, want to do C. To build the confidence to continue asking your doctor questions, you'll mentally remind yourself that, yes, doctors are on tighter schedules now, but your doctor has an obligation to listen to you and answer your questions. Remind yourself that it takes extra energy to be assertive, but it will pay off in the long run. If you have trouble doing this for yourself, consider how you would handle the situation if someone you love—such as your spouse—needed this information. Sometimes it is easier for us to advocate or talk on the behalf of others, than for ourselves.

In this situation, you need to stay calm. Let your doctor know that you do not understand. Ask if he has patient education materials about the medication. These materials often explain things in a less technical way. We all learn in different ways. Some learn by hearing, some by seeing, and others by reading. So ask if you can have something in writing that you can take home with you.

USE EFFECTIVE BODY LANGUAGE

YOUR TONE OF voice, facial expression, posture, and gestures can help you get your points across more clearly. When talking with your physicians, do the following:

Look him or her in the eyes. If you are nervous or not good at eye contact, look through, beyond, or just above his eyes, but keep your eyes on him somewhere!

Sit up. Try not to slump your shoulders. Lean forward as you talk. Look as though you mean what you are saying and you are convinced in your thoughts.

Use your hands. Gestures can not only help you feel more comfortable standing your ground, they can also help you more strongly make a point.

Look serious. Many people tend to smile or laugh inappropriately with they feel embarrassed or on the spot. If you are talking about something serious, try to keep a serious expression on your face. Match your facial expression with your spoken words.

ADDITIONAL COMMUNICATION STRATEGIES

IN ADDITION TO monitoring your thoughts and practicing before your visit, try the following communication strategies:

Determine short-term and longer-term goals for care. What are your goals for treatment besides the obvious one: staying alive? Do you want to stay as functional as possible throughout your care, no matter what? Are a few months of being wiped out from treatment worth it for a while? What kind of flexibility do you have in your life and job? Write down your answers and take your replies with you to the doctor's appointment. If you can't actually voice your needs, just hand it over and let your doctor read it. Ask your doctor for his or her views and what he or she would suggest. Mail a copy of your list to the office before your appointment and bring another copy with you.

Don't assume you know what your doctor is thinking. None of us has the ability to read minds. Don't misinterpret your doctor's quick speech as an indication that he or she isn't willing to listen to you. Your physician is probably trying to do his or her best and doesn't realize he or she is bombarding you with statistics that make your head spin. Also many patients worry they will offend their physicians by asking for a second opinion or a referral to a specialist, yet physicians are used to such requests and generally do not take them personally. Do not worry about your doctor's feelings. Keep the focus on your health. Give your doctor the benefit of the doubt first by assertively addressing the problem. Tell your doctor what he or she does that seems to confuse you. Ask your doctor to talk more slowly, explain things in plain English, or repeat the reason for the recommendation. If this type of frank discussion does not improve the situation, then it may be time to find a new doctor!

Monitor your feelings. You may feel angry for all sorts of reasons, but try not to take this out on your doctor. You may be really tired and feel pretty passive that day, but you really want to be part of decision-making regarding your care. Think about the points you want to get across before the visit.

Speak your mind regarding your care. Tell the doctor how you really feel about a certain side effects or clinical effects that you read about, regarding a certain treatment that he or she would like to try with you. Ask about various treatments and their clinical effects. If your doctor prescribes medication that makes you feel tired and listless, speak up. Say it, if you are open to trying a different drug or a different dose. Realize that there is not one optimal dose for all people. This is part of the art in medicine, and only with your feedback will your doctor be able to adjust the dosage that's right for you.

Repeat yourself. Your physician may have many things on his or her mind as he or she examines and listens to you, and may not actually hear everything that you say. So repeat yourself. Also, if you are generally shy or have gotten into a more passive mode since your illness, you may not express yourself clearly the first time you try to get a point across. On your second time through, you'll generally deliver a clearer message. Speak up, and don't let a point that is important to you slide by—paraphrase or repeat it until you receive a response.

Take along some backup. Ask a family member or friend to come to the appointment with you. If you don't speak up about the problem you wish to address, your friend or family member should prompt you—or even do it for you.

Get help. If you have found that you get really nervous before these doctor visits or you have problems getting your intentions heard, learn some relaxation or assertiveness techniques or consider alternative medicine techniques, such as acupuncture, to help you relax. Consult chapter 6 for strategies to enable relaxation. Choose a method that will help you to lower your stress overall and before your appointment, and stay relaxed and focused during your visit.

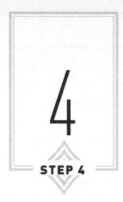

STEP 4

Form a Strong Support Team

UNTIL NOW, WE have focused mainly on your health and health care. Now, it's time to explore your quality of life, that overall sense of well-being and enjoyment of life. In the coming chapters, we will explore numerous ways to improve your outlook on life. For example, in chapter 5, you'll discover ways to improve your lifestyle. In chapter 6, you'll find strategies to bolster your emotional health.

In this chapter, you'll learn about one of the most important indicators of your quality of life—your relationships with others. When you were undergoing major treatment for cancer, you may have had more support than you knew what to do with. Family members accompanied you to every doctor's appointment, test, and procedure. Friends cooked meals, cut the grass, trimmed the hedges, and more. Neighbors watched the kids. Co-workers sent flowers, cards, and motivating letters and e-mails. Your physicians spent lots of time with you, explaining every option in great detail.

Then, you finished your last radiation or chemotherapy session. For a time, things may still have run smoothly. Perhaps family and friends threw you a party or went to a series of follow-up visits with you. Those friends from church and other community organizations continued to check in. But as the days, weeks, and months began to click by, your support team began to dry up. The church and civic community got involved in other projects. Your spouse, children, and close friends returned to their long-neglected personal lives and interests. Your doctor's appointments became fewer and farther between, and you were left to fend for yourself. For your support team, life was returning to normal. That is expected, after all.

Yet, as you know, life after cancer is still hard. You now must deal with the side effects of your treatments. These can include everything from premature menopause to sexual dysfunction. You must confront those mounting medical bills. You may battle with your employer or your health insurance company. You may not be able to complete daily tasks, such as house or yard work, at all or at the pace you want to.

And, possibly most important, like all human beings, you need a group of people that you feel close to, to listen to your feelings and help you to feel loved. Indeed, study after study points to what has now become an indisputable fact: social support makes us healthier and extends our lives. One study on women with metastatic breast cancer found that, the larger the women's support system, the better their mood and the lower their stress levels. Also, research shows that social support is most critical when you need to deal with stressful experiences—such as those you might encounter during cancer survival. In these cases, social support helps prevent your immunity from taking a nosedive.

Close ties to family, friends, and the community not only instill a reason for being, they also provide a steady and large network of people who can lend a hand—or a shoulder—during tough times. This reduces stress, which, as you will learn in chapter 6, is critical to optimizing your survival.

Here's the good news. No matter what your current level of support, you can take a few simple steps to improve it. Doing so will greatly improve your health and quality of life. Consider this: social support can help you to find the motivation and willpower to improve lifestyle habits. Having a hard time eating more vegetables? Your spouse and other family members can make sure they are available to you at every opportunity. Here are some ways in which others may be supportive:

- Your support team can help you brainstorm ways to improve your health and make decisions. If you're struggling with an important health-care decision, your support team can help you weigh your pros and cons and do some research for you.
- When you feel down or start focusing on the past, members of your support team can help you to snap out of it. You might lean on your faith to bolster your spirits or call a friend when you are not feeling yourself.
- When you need help with physical tasks—such as cutting the grass,

basic housework, or navigating that pile of bills—your support team can lighten the load.

- Members of your support team can accompany you to important tests and doctor's visits. The presence of a loved one or friend can help keep you calm—especially during repeat diagnostic tests. Your friend or loved one can also take notes during the visit, to ensure you both remember your doctor's advice more accurately.

- Supportive co-workers can take on tasks for you that you no longer can handle due to treatment-induced symptoms, such as low energy levels. They can also help you to talk out frustrations you have about work or your supervisor, allowing you to shed some steam.

- A support team can also help you keep life in perspective. Family, friends, support groups, spiritual communities, and anonymous online chat rooms can all give you support. You can also look inside for support by using practical spiritual approaches.

- All told, your team can help you embrace life to the fullest, encouraging you to find new meaning for each day and search for the answers to lingering issues. You can celebrate the positive experiences in life with members of your team, too.

- In the following pages, you'll discover how to maximize support in all areas of your life—family, friends, co-workers, and spiritual communities. You'll learn how to not only build a large support team, but also a strong one, whose members can help you to optimize your survival without burning themselves out in the process.

GETTING THE SUPPORT YOU NEED

USE THIS SIMPLE self-assessment to determine whether you need to improve your social network. According to research, cancer survivors benefit from three types of support: emotional, instrumental, and informational. Emotional support stems from people who are closest to you, such as a spouse, a partner, your brothers or sisters, and/or your adult sons or daughters. Good emotional support, particularly from your closest family or friends, can help you feel better about yourself. Instrumental support includes the hands-on help you may need, such as someone to drive you to an appointment, help you cook or clean, or assist with some tasks at work. Informational support refers to your ability to get the right type of information you need to guide your decisions regarding health, health care, and quality-of-life questions that crop up.

To assess your current level of support, circle Yes or No for each of the following questions.

GETTING THE SUPPORT YOU NEED		
EMOTIONAL SUPPORT (People who help you feel positive)		
A.1.	I feel as if my family is "there for me."	Yes	No
A.2.	My family listens to me.	Yes	No
A.3.	My family reassures me.	Yes	No
A.4.	I feel comforted when I talk to my family.	Yes	No
A.5.	I feel loved by my family.	Yes	No
INSTRUMENTAL SUPPORT (People who help to make life easier)		
B.1.	I can get help with housework/yard work when I need it.	Yes	No
B.2.	People make meals for me if I need them.	Yes	No
B.3.	If I need a ride for any reason, I can get someone to drive me.	Yes	No
B.4.	If I need money, I have friends or family who can loan it to me.	Yes	No
B.5.	If I need someone to watch the kids, I have a trustworthy person do that.	Yes	No
INFORMATIONAL SUPPORT (People who help you find the knowledge you need to move forward)		
C.1.	Doctors provide me with the timely medical information I need.	Yes	No
C.2.	Doctors encourage me with my self-care decisions.	Yes	No
C.3.	I receive a helpful amount of advice/information from my family.	Yes	No
C.4.	I feel my family approves of my ongoing life decisions.	Yes	No
C.5.	When I have a problem, I can turn to someone I trust to help me solve it.	Yes	No

What your answers mean

Look over your answers. Which of the three sections have the most no answers? The more No's you circle, the less support you have in a given area. Consult each area below to see how to strengthen your support network, focusing on the area with the most no answers first.

Your emotional support system: Talk to your family members, letting them know how much you appreciate them. Tell them that you would like everyone to express their feelings rather than keeping them to themselves! Also, you may benefit from seeing a counselor to help you communicate better with certain family members. Remember, they are going through a change, too. Even though they care about you a lot, the cancer experience may cloud their world, making it difficult for loved ones to accurately hear what you are saying. Try to make family members as comfortable about sharing their feelings as possible. Children especially may hide their true feelings from you out of a desire to protect *your* feelings. Tell your family that you can "take it" and want open and honest communication—negative or positive. For more advice on communicating with your family, see Strengthening Family Support on page 84.

Your instrumental support system: Think about resources you may have available to you but, for whatever reasons, you have not tapped into yet. Accepting help is not easy for a lot of people, but using help can make your life easier and improve its quality. For example, if you could find an affordable housekeeping service, you may find more physical energy to get out of your house and do some things with friends that you did not feel up to because you were wasting your energy on housework. Contact organizations such as the American Cancer Society, your neighborhood township office, or even your place of worship for additional possible sources of support.

Your informational support system: Medical professionals provide the information that people most trust, so lean heavily on your physician and other medical professionals. Ask the nurses and physician assistants at your physician's office to explain treatments, medications, and tests. If you are unclear about your physician's suggestions, ask your doctor or support staff for a handout or some other type of written instructions. In addition to your physician and physician's staff, lean on your pharmacist as well. Few people ask questions when they fill prescriptions, but they should! Your pharmacist can help alert you to possible drug interactions, explain possible side effects of over-the-counter medicines and supplements, and may even be able to help reduce your prescription drug bill by suggesting generic alternatives to brand medications prescribed by your doctor.

STRENGTHENING FAMILY SUPPORT

CANCER HAS A perverse way of reminding family members of their importance to one another—bringing everyone closer emotionally—as it simultaneously strains family relationships. For example, after my cancer diagnosis, I generally grew closer to my family, which provided me with a great deal of support during and after the initial illness. That said, I still have to work at it. Sometimes I don't have the energy to go out or stay somewhere once I'm out. I, of course, feel bad about this, as I know my fatigue often causes my wife or kids to forgo social situations or cut them short before *they* are ready. At times I also feel as if everyone expects me to be just like I was before. I do the best I can, trying to communicate clearly about how I feel and what I think I can and cannot do, but it takes effort and it doesn't always make a difference.

> ### *Survivor Stat*
>
> A STUDY OF ovarian cancer patients determined that women with higher levels of "social attachment" had lower blood levels of interleukin 6. High levels of this pro-inflammatory cytokine has been linked with increased risk of cancer metastasis (cancer spreading to other organs).

The effort, of course, is well worth it. Family and friends greatly influence our self-esteem. Their support not only makes us feel loved, it can help to reduce stress.

According to research conducted on cancer survivors, family and friends are supportive most of the time, but not completely supportive at other times. In fact, this research shows they sometimes undermine your feelings of control and self-esteem by doing the following:

Criticizing the way you handle your survivorship: Family and friends mean well when they say things like, "Why are you down today? You should be thankful that you are doing so well," or " Stop thinking about it. I could die today just crossing the street," or "Why don't you just think about the cancer only on the day you come back for a follow-up." "Don't worry about getting it all completed. Take it one day at a time." People really do want to help but often simply don't know what to say. Unfortunately, such comments aren't always helpful. You already know these things. It's like standing behind a plumber who has come to fix your toilet and, every few minutes saying, "The toilet is still broken." Yes, that's true, but your comments don't help the plumber fix your toilet any faster!

Instead of suggesting that the approach you are taking to your own survivorship needs to be changed, ask family and friends to *listen*. Tell them that you understand their desire to help, but that they could be even more helpful if they listened to and just acknowledged your feelings. Explain that you don't need them to try to cheer you up or always fix the situation. They will feel relieved, too.

Physically avoiding you: Some friends or even family members may feel uncomfortable talking with you about your illness. They worry that they will say something to upset you, so they respond by saying nothing at all. Such people may even avoid you, making excuses to get off the phone or bail out of dinner appointments. Others who spent a lot of time helping you battle cancer may now be burned out and need more time alone. Either way, you're left to wonder if you somehow have offended this person.

Be proactive in these situations. Talk with the person, explaining that you sense a certain level of discomfort. Ask whether you've done or said something to make him or her uncomfortable around you. Ask point blank, "It seems as if you are avoiding me. Why is that?" Often this simple conversation will serve as an icebreaker, helping your friend or family member to realize that he or she *can* comfortably talk with you about cancer (or anything else for that matter).

Minimizing what you are experiencing: In response to your comments about your poor memory, fatigue, or other treatment-induced symptoms, some friends and family members may try to make you feel better by making statements such as, "You are just getting older, that's why you can't remember things," or "I can't do that, either." Explain how these comments affect you. Say "You could help me even more if you would simply acknowledge what I am going through and work with me to find some possible solutions."

Avoiding discussions about cancer or related problems: Let's say you and your family are watching TV. A news special comes on about cancer. You say, "Yes, that's just like I feel," or "I have that problem, too," but no one from your family responds. Or let's say you're too tired to go to a social event and you try to explain why you'd rather stay home, but your family ignores you, proceeding as if everything is okay. Sometimes, cancer survival strains relationships because you have been through a battle and you are tired. You often emerge a different person, seeing the world in a new way. Yet your spouse, family, and friends have not gone through it exactly the way you did and they have not emerged with some new sense of meaning and fullness. Remember this: you need to be very clear in your communications indicating your view. You also need to realize that sometimes your family and friends either don't want to see you as different because it is frightening or they simply can't understand your actions. The thing to do is to try to understand that families and friends are cancer survivors, too.

Walk in Their Shoes

Talk directly to your family and friends. Family and friends have feelings and thoughts about the cancer, so hear them out and try to understand their point of view. Usually, most people do not undermine you on purpose. They may do so based on their own feelings of helplessness, uncertainty, loss, or personal stress. Remember that many family members and friends have been there for you through the worst. They drove you to your treatments and stayed and talked with you during chemo or helped you pick up or organize your medication. They shopped with you for wigs and scarves, and jotted down notes at your doctors' appointments. Many support people get tired after a while. They may lose patience easily or simply want to get on with their own lives.

Also, remember that family and friends may mistakenly think that the battle is over for you. You beat the cancer, right? As a result, they may feel that you no longer need their support. You may need to remind them that survivorship is a continuous journey.

To get a better idea of how to accomplish this type of open communication when focusing on cancer, let's take a look at two common, related problems that many survivors tell me they face with their families—along with how open, honest communication can help solve the issues. Both of these examples center on how your family can help support you when it comes to gathering information about health. Often survivors tell me that they'd like their families to help them with this because it can get overwhelming, but they run into one of the following common obstacles:

- Family members tend to provide information or opinions that are just too confusing or that are just not helpful. These family members often provide the survivor with the latest tip they found while surfing the Internet or reading the newspaper or watching TV which may not be applicable to them or may not help generate information related to their specific concern or problem.

- Family members don't want to spend the time to help search for potential solutions to a nagging problem given other priorities saying they are too busy to help and that's what doctors are for anyway. As we know we often need to explore options on our own rather than totally relying on health professionals.

Let's first take a look at how you might solve the first issue. In this scenario, you would simply thank them for their concern, explaining that you and your doctors are keeping you on top of the situation.

The second scenario requires a little more finesse on your part, because you are essentially trying to get your spouse or kids to do something they don't feel is that important. It's much like those battles you waged to get your kids to eat their broccoli. You were right, but you couldn't force them to listen to you. In this case, it might be worth backing down. Of course, explain *why* you want and need the help, along with how your partner's or kid's refusal makes you feel. Ask your family members why they don't want to help. Really listen to their reply. To encourage yourself to listen—rather than formulate your rebuttal as they speak—take notes and repeat back to them what you think you heard them say. Work out a compromise. If, after this candid discussion and compromise things don't work out, make your peace with the situation. You did the best you could do. The point of all this is the need to keep your focus on the process—the open, honest communication within the family or among friends—and not on the outcome. After all, the more often you have such discussions, the closer you can grow—even if you don't initially get the result you want.

When building your support team, remember that open, honest communication goes both ways. You can't sit back and wait for your family and friends to change. You need to be proactive. Most important, you must be just as open and honest that you expect from others. I've counseled many cancer survivors over the years. Many of them keep their real feelings about cancer to themselves. I know it's not easy talking about fears. Who wants to burden someone with the anxiety you feel about something at work, for example, when you have bigger concerns, like how long you really are going to live? After all, who wants to hear negative things all the time? Also, when everyone around you is trying to cheer you up and encourage you to think positively, it's hard to open up and let your fears, frustrations, or despair spill out.

For example, a few years ago, I counseled Jim, a thirty-five-year-old cancer survivor who initially came to me for anxiety and pain he experienced. After talking with him about his situation, I realized that the pain and anxiety stemmed from a problem within the family. Jim's cancer had recurred, yet this man could not bring himself to tell his wife or children. When I spoke with his wife Sally, I learned that she suspected the cancer had returned and was probably worse. On several occasions she had tried to talk to him about it, but he did not want to discuss it with her.

Over a series of sessions with Jim and Sally, Jim began to feel more comfortable discussing with Sally some of his deepest fears. Eventually he told his wife about his cancer recurrence and his expected outcome. He felt relieved. Sally and his kids were much more understanding than he had imagined. Together he and his wife formed a number of possible scenarios for the future such as how the children will be schooled (they were home schooled and Sally would need to work), how the family will handle financial concerns, and how holidays would be spent. After these family discussions, he and his wife and children felt closer. They also supported him by letting him know that they will be okay in the long run, assuring him they can do all sorts of things around the house that he traditionally had handled, such as taking out garbage, changing lightbulbs, doing lawn work, and shoveling snow. Not only did he feel better emotionally, he was better able to manage the pain he experienced.

Survivor Stat

A **RECENT STUDY** of colorectal, breast, and prostate cancer survivors found that families able to interact with each other openly and express feelings directly, and who worked to effectively solve problems related to cancer survivorship, report much lower levels of depression. The study also reported that when the family talked about the survivor's symptoms or other problems, feelings of anxiety were lower too. Clearly, the way in which a family reacts to the cancer experience influences everyone's mood and day to quality of life in the family.

How Children Cope

In an interesting study, parents diagnosed with cancer thought that their children were adjusting to their cancer diagnosis quite well, with no apparent emotional or behavioral problems. Yet, when researchers studied questionnaires filled out by these children, they found that teenage girls

Emotional Support: From the Heart

YOUR FAMILY CAN provide a type of support that you'll be hard pressed to develop in many other areas of your life. You certainly don't have to be a cancer survivor to celebrate births of children and grandchildren, high school graduations, and other milestones. Nor do you have to have survived cancer to appreciate occasional phone calls from grown children "just to talk" or handwritten notes for special occasions. Yet, when you have survived cancer, these small gestures can really keep you going. Below you will find some examples of cards that survivors have shown me over the years, cards they received from family members at a critical time in their survivorship journey. These statements don't mention cancer specifically, but they make a difference in whether you just plug along or really strive to thrive.

I love spending time with you. Mommy told me all about the boat and I can't wait to come on it! She also said you play the guitar. Can you play and sing Raffi songs for me? I am so lucky to have you as my papa. I love you.

I love you so much! You have been a wonderful mother all my life. I still remember all the fun times and trips the two of us took together when I was a child and now that I have a son we will continue to spend lots of time together.

Thank you for all you do for our family. You are always strong and give us all inspiration to never give up. I love you so much.

Thank you for being such a great father to our children! They all love and cherish you so much! I love you with all my heart.

actually had high levels of anxiety and depression. This is worrisome considering their parents thought they were adjusting just fine!

Some of the concerns children and other family members can experience include:

Worry and fear: Children may feel shock, disbelief, numbness, powerlessness, and intense feelings of sadness about your diagnoses and treatment. Many children report that even months or years after a parent's diagnoses, they "can't believe it happened." Some during a parent's survivorship say they wish they could do more to help. This is why it's so important to include your children in your support team. Although you don't want to overburden them with tasks and chores, let them know how they can help you. Also, try not to hide the facts of your health from them. The more children know and understand, the less fear they will carry around with them.

> ### Survivor Stat
>
> NINETY-THREE PERCENT of adult daughters of cancer survivors reported at least one positive change in the aftermath of their parent's cancer.

A desire to protect: Children and spouses may hide their feelings about your battle with cancer, in an attempt to ease your burden. They may feel you are already sad, frustrated, or depressed as it is and don't want to add to it by telling you about their feelings. It's hard to walk on eggshells day in and day out, so do your best to remove the shells from the path of your family members! Explain to your spouse and children that there's nothing they can tell you that will upset you even more. Tell them that, while keeping their feelings to themselves may have helped to keep you calm during your treatment, you now want to grow closer as a family. Explain that you are stronger now than you were at the beginning of your cancer journey.

A struggle to adjust to the new you: Even if you don't talk about the new you, your spouse and kids know that things have changed. Many children respond by trying to find out everything they can about cancer. They choose cancer as research topics at school, for example. They also notice your limitations. They can tell if you become frustrated easily, can't remember things as well as you used to, and whether you feel fatigued. So not talking about it doesn't hide it! You can help your family adjust to the new you more quickly by being open and honest about your challenges. For example, hold a family meeting to talk about who needs to do what to get things done around the house.

Communicating Your Needs

Even if you have kept your feelings to yourself for quite a long time, you can still open up to your family and strengthen this supportive tie. The degree to which you do this really depends on you, the stage of your survival, and your family's level of interest and cooperation. Use the following tips.

- Talk about the problems and challenges that crop up. For example, when I do not want to join in family events outside the house, but would rather sit at home and relax or read, I mention this to the rest of the family; everyone knows that it's not something that is personal (i.e., that don't want to be with them), but rather is a consequence of how I feel physically at the time. Also, we have all learned to laugh about my cognitive challenges rather than having long drawn out discussions about them. This type of reaction reassures me that my family understands.
- Let your kids know how much you love them and how proud you are of them. This, of course, is important in any family, but particularly after a battle with cancer. During your major treatments, you may not have spent as much time with your kids. You may have missed some Little League games and school plays. Make up for that now by showing your kids just how much you care about them.
- Ask your children about fun things they would like to do with you—and do them. Again, it's important for all families to do this, but even more so after a battle with cancer. If anything, cancer has taught you that time is precious. Make the most of it!
- Ask them how they feel about things. Listen to their answers without comment. Don't judge their feelings. Acknowledge them.
- Point out positive aspects of your health to your children. Let your children know, for example, that you are feeling stronger (if you are) or that you are now able to do something you couldn't a while ago. This shows them that you are able to do things for yourself and reduces pressure on them so they don't feel the need to protect you.
- Make it clear what you would like your spouse and children to do to help out in the home now that you can't do as much. Discuss options with them rather than dictating a long chore list.
- Spend one-on-one time with each of your children, your spouse, and your friends.

- Try to create a routine that allows the family to talk about concerns and everyday matters. While this is hard to do with everyone's schedules for many families, dinner hour still works best. With everyone seated at the table and the TV off, talk about possible challenges that you and other family members face, and then use the problem-solving technique outlined in chapter 2 to come up with possible solutions.

- Take as many steps as possible to get back to a precancer relationship with your children. You can't sweep your battle with cancer under the rug. You must address it. Yet, there's a fine line between addressing challenges and solving problems and wallowing in them.

- Do things together as a family. This is especially important if you run into a brick wall when trying to communicate your needs with your spouse and kids. Sometimes family members simply don't want to talk. They don't like to share or listen to feelings. They dig in their heels. In this case, grow closer through your actions rather than your words. Take walks, go shopping or to the movies together or whatever they suggest.

Your Children and Your Cancer

CANCER AND CANCER survival affects our kids greatly, adding another layer of stress. I had the opportunity to read a personal narrative that Erica, my youngest daughter, wrote for an English class during her senior year in high school, three years after my diagnosis. It highlights many of her thoughts regarding our battle with cancer. The following essay helped me better understand Erica's reaction to this event, allowing me to realize how stressful this was for her, too.

> Sometimes waiting can be the most difficult task of all. In June of 2002, waiting seemed to be the only constant in my life. On a day when people were carelessly enjoying the gorgeous summer weather, my family and I were inside a dark and unwelcoming hospital waiting for my dad's neurosurgeon to finish his operation. My sister sat by my side as we waited, what felt like an eternity, for my dad to come out of brain surgery. With his arm around our mom, my brother tried to lighten the mood with his humor. We sat as a family of four, waiting for our fifth member to return to us healthy

and alive. Tears of fear and love slowly streamed down my face and landed on the stuffed dog my dad had given me years before. I held onto it for strength and courage as I thought of my dad and wondered, "Why him? Why did such a good man have to suffer from a brain tumor?" These questions will forever be unanswered.

After hours of waiting, my dad's doctor told us that Dad had made it through the risky surgery and we could finally go visit him. It wasn't until I saw him that I realized the severity of his illness. My dad lay in a hospital bed with his head bandaged, the blood slowly beginning to seep through the once pure white gauze. Only a thin hanging sheet separated dad from the man screaming for his life in the bed next to him. My dad slept soundly. A nurse told my family that he was doing great, but it didn't look that way.

My dad has always been the glue that holds my family together; he gives the best advice, helps with homework and always knows how to cheer me up. It was hard to understand that a man, who was so full of life just a day before, could now appear so helpless. It took three long weeks of waiting for the doctors to come to a conclusion about the tumor. It was malignant. The once unimaginable came to reality for my dad and the whole family: cancer. Over the next two years, my dad underwent extensive radiation and chemotherapy. He never lost hope and never for a second made me think he wouldn't make it through the seemingly never-ending road to recovery.

Each year since my dad's diagnosis I have participated in the Race for Hope, a run to support research for the treatment of brain tumors. This year I ran with men, women, and children who I had never met, yet who were all running for the same cause. I was proud to be wearing the words, "I am honoring the survival of my dad, Michael Feuerstein," on my shirt as I ran. With each stride I was reminded of the painful memories of waiting, memories I still try so hard to put behind me. During the race I felt both physically and emotionally drained, but I never let myself slow down. My dad never gave up, so I didn't, either. He will forever be my inspiration and hero in everything I do. My dad's cancer has showed me how fortunate I am to have him healthy again, and to appreciate not only the people close to me, but life itself.

YOUR SURVIVORSHIP

Up to now I have focused on the family who wants to help out; unfortunately, not all families do or can. For all sorts of reasons, families fall into old patterns of relating to others and having cancer doesn't change that. If a family member was not supportive of others before the illness it is very unlikely that things are going to change. In fact, it is far healthier in such a situation to move forward without attempting to pursue something that may create even more stress in your life. Rather than calling on a hesistant family member, you might want to call on a friend, coworker, someone in your religious community, or a support group. Research indicates that external support is crucial to survivorship. Support from family and/or friends can help in many ways and survivors should seek it when and wherever possible. Who comprises your support team is personal and up to each of you. There is no ideal way to generate support but it is important to survivorship.

WORKPLACE SUPPORT

In addition to your family, you can also find support at work. Co-workers can help you maximize your quality of life by going to lunch with you or taking walks with you at lunch so you can get the exercise you need to stay fit. Co-workers can also serve as sounding boards, helping you to shed some of your anger and frustration. Possibly, most important, your co-workers can help you to solve problems you might encounter at work—even problems that you encounter with other co-workers! Although you may naturally feel close to some co-workers and not mind talking about your battle with cancer with them, you might not necessary feel close to all of them. Some of these fellow workers may not understand what you have gone through and how things may have changed for you. Maybe you used to be totally involved in your work, and now, for you, it is just a job. Maybe you don't have as much energy as you did before your treatment. Maybe your perspective on work or other things in life are different now. Whatever the reasons, your co-workers will notice the new you and wonder what the heck happened.

If comments or persistent questions from these fellow workers begin to drag you down, lean on your workplace support team for help. One of these supportive co-workers can talk to the others, explaining what you

How to Deal with Busybodies

GENERALLY, PEOPLE MEAN well, but persistent questioning from nosy co-workers can not only become awkward but downright annoying. So, before you return to work, think about some of the types of questions they may ask and formulate answers in your mind so you are more prepared when the questions to come up.

Common questions co-workers ask include:

- What's it like to have cancer?
- Is it hard for you to work?
- Did your insurance pay for everything?
- How much does this type of thing cost?
- What was the radiation and chemotherapy like?
- How is your family taking it?
- What's your health situation now?
- Do you still have cancer?

People are curious. Some ask thoughtless questions, others don't know what to say. Some people will want to share stories of their friends, family, or other loved ones who had similar situations, while still others may ignore or try to normalize the situation to help keep themselves at ease. Your attitude will lead the way much of the time. A simple response of "Fine, thank you for your concern" is a nice way to answer many questions. Then change the subject, if you need to, or open it up if you want to talk to this colleague a bit more. While this situation may seen awkward at first, it can be handled as you would any other personal conversation.

are going through and asking them to put a lid on their questions—at least until you get back on your feet and feel ready to deal with them.

So, find a few people you can count on to talk to, people who you feel you can discuss some of your concerns with. Use them as a sounding board or to help you generate ideas of how you can approach problems at work. For example, you might ask a co-worker to help you solve a problem you've encountered since you've returned to work. Go through the problem-solving technique outlined in chapter 2 together. Your co-worker may be able to help you better define the problem and generate possible solutions. A side benefit to such a structured interaction is that you can express some of your frustration about previous ineffective approaches you've used to solve the problem.

Let's say you forgot to tell your boss about an important meeting that you could not attend because of a doctor's appointment. Or, you get into an argument with your supervisor because it takes longer for you to get things done now and she leaves with a negative view of your abilities. You might head to a co-workers office to blow off some steam and when composed, work on defining the problem, and generate some ways to effectively solve it.

Much of the communication with your colleagues will depend on the type of relationship you had with them before you found out you had cancer. Provide only the information about your health that you feel comfortable sharing, and share that information only with people in your support team.

SPIRITUAL SUPPORT

FOR THOUSANDS OF years, spirituality has been linked to healing and a sense of well-being. It doesn't matter whether you go to a church, synagogue, mosque, or temple. The effect is often the same. Spiritual support can improve your optimism and hope, reduce distress, and may even help you finally become at peace with the unknown. Many survivors tell me that becoming more spiritual helped them increase their feelings of control and their quality of life.

According to one study, actively expressing religious beliefs by going to a place of worship, praying, or performing some other personal religious activity helps bolster self-esteem and well-being. Patients who had a greater sense of well-being were better able to cope with cancer over the long term and find meaning in the cancer experience. The routine of religious holidays can provide a structure for some people.

Many studies have uncovered benefits of prayer and faith, showing, for example, that heart bypass patients who were prayed over were more likely to live than bypass patients who were not prayed over. Although this area remains controversial in terms of the effectiveness of spirituality on health some of these findings include the following:

- Of 734 elderly Danish men and women, those who were affiliated with a place of worship tended to live longer than those who did not have a religious affiliation.
- In a study of 150 people who cared for loved ones with Alzheimer's disease, researchers determined that caregivers who scored higher on a spiritual well-being questionnaire (indicating strong religious or spiritual beliefs) felt less burdened by their caregiving responsibilities than caregivers who scored low on the same questionnaire.

So, if you believe that prayer, meditation, or attending a religious service helps *you* feel better . . . then do it. Research shows it works.

That said, be careful about attributing too much to the healing power of religion. For example, one night recently I went to a support group for people with brain tumors, in Washington, D.C. A new member of the group showed up. Joe was a very gentle and positive, and many group members quickly welcomed him. Joe had been diagnosed with a major type of malignant brain tumor and had undergone radiation and a few months of chemotherapy. Joe told an incredible story. He had dreamt one night that angels came and replaced his cancer-ridden brain with a new brain that was healthy. A few days after dreaming this scenario, he had an MRI. The scan found no evidence of cancer. Because of his strong religious beliefs, he felt God had intervened in his life and had cured him of the cancer. As a result, he halted his chemotherapy treatments.

At first, I was of course amazed, as were other group members. I believe strongly in the healing power of religion. At the same time, as a scientist, clinician, and survivor, I felt the implications of his actions could be fatal. The change in this man's tumor status could just as well, scientifically speaking, been a result of his radiation and chemotherapy treatments—treatment he had discontinued.

Why do I belabor this? What is the message? Yes, it is important to believe in a higher power, but it's just as important to remain realistic. Use spiritual belief and support *in conjunction* with regular medical care and not *instead of* it! It's simply not wise to discontinue a course of evidence-based medical treatment just because you now believe your God has intervened in your situation.

Please don't misunderstand me. I'm not knocking religion or the affect of a higher power. I'm only saying that you shouldn't use it as a substitute for conventional medicine. Use your religious community as a place for physical and mental support. Allow your spirituality to fortify you both mentally and physically. But don't make the mistake of firing your doctor because of it.

Test Your Spiritual IQ

You can't judge your level of spiritual support as easily as you can assess your level of exercise or healthy eating habits. Simply placing an *x* on your calendar every time you go to church or counting up your number of spiritual or religious friends won't necessarily make you see the meaning of your life and at feel peace.

The following quiz, however, can help. It can help you to find out whether you could use more spiritual support in your life. There are no right or wrong answers to these questions. I've included this self-assessment so you can reflect on your beliefs. Your answers will show you whether you are struggling with these key areas of life.

	TEST YOUR SPIRITUAL IQ		
	SPiRITUAL WELL-BEING	**YES**	**NO**
1.	I feel peaceful.		
2.	I have a reason for living.		
3.	My life has been productive.		
4.	I have trouble feeling peace of mind.		
5.	I feel a sense of purpose in my life.		
6.	I am able to reach deep down into myself for comfort.		
7.	I feel a sense of harmony within myself.		
8.	My life lacks meaning and purpose.		
9.	I find comfort in my faith or spiritual beliefs.		
10.	I find strength in my faith or spiritual beliefs.		
11.	My illness has strengthened my faith or spiritual beliefs.		
12.	I know that whatever happens with my illness, things will be okay.		

These questions have been adapted using the Yes and No answers with permission from the Functional Assessment of Chronic Illness Therapy (FACIT) spiritual well-being scale (copyright, FACIT.org). See www.facit.org for more information.

Okay, now that you've answered the questions, let's take a look at what your answers mean. Take a look at the following three areas describing a range of attitudes. These descriptions are not a fortune-teller's response about your personal spiritual beliefs. They are summaries of how your answers relate to your level of spirituality and, in turn, your potential well-being.

> **AREA 1: No regrets, looking forward. If you checked Yes to questions 1, 2, 3, 5, 6, 7:** Things are going well for you. You feel good about the life you lived and are now living. You have a sense of purpose and inner calmness.
> **AREA 2: Constructive perspectives. If you checked Yes to questions: 5, 6, 7, 9, 10, 11, 12:** You indicate that you're able to accept what has transpired over the time since your diagnosis. You have a focus in your life and find that you can search for meaning within yourself. You also find comfort and strength in your spiritual beliefs.
> **AREA 3: Time to move forward. If you checked No to questions 4 or 8 or both:** You report a general sense of uneasiness. These feelings can be common experiences when threatened with something like cancer.

So what do you do if you answered no where you could have answered yes? This doesn't mean you've failed Spirituality 101. It only means that you could create a greater sense of meaning and comfort in your life. Keep reading to find out initial steps on how to do just that.

Infuse Your Life with Meaning

If after taking the self-assessment you decide that you'd like to create a greater sense of meaning and peace in your life, consider sitting down with a minister, priest, rabbi, or other type of spiritual counselor and talking about that issue. You can also attend religious services on a regular basis or become involved in some formal activity with a religious focus.

If formal religion is not your thing, consider the ways the following cancer survivors have used spirituality to reduce stress and increase their sense of purpose in life:

■ Terry, a breast cancer survivor, was brought up in a religious environment as a child. Yet, she told me that she "really did not actively participate in religion as an adult." That said, since her diagnosis and treatment, she prays daily for "strength, health, and that the cancer does not recur."

While at times she gets down and "her mind starts working," she does "shake it off" and move on to more positive thoughts.

- Bob, a survivor of spinal cord cancer, told me that he developed a "spiritual connection" after his cancer diagnosis. He believes that this spirituality helps him relax and keeps him going. This spiritual force helps him move forward in his life, keeps him physically active, and helps his mood. He believes that the survival statistics the doctors tell him about provide only "one perspective of who gets through this." He volunteers, helping others with cancer to gain a spiritual perspective. This experience has helped mold and maintain his positive, can-do attitude.

- Jim, a survivor of Hodgkin's lymphoma, was brought up going to church, but admitted to me that he only turns to prayer when he is sick. He is fine with this, although he, of course, feels a little sheepish talking about it. Praying, he says, calms him and helps him feel better overall.

In addition to prayer and a belief in something larger than yourself, you can also look into something called "practical spirituality." What is practical spirituality? A medical scientist and psychologist, describes it this way: "Each one of us has the right to happiness and peace. As we move toward these qualities within ourselves, we become more joyful, creative, and healthy. The attitudes of patience, kindness, gratitude, understanding, and compassion naturally evolve, and we become generators of peace in our homes and workplaces."

Practical spirituality provides specific techniques to help you generate these meaningful qualities within yourself. It teaches you to recognize certain patterns to your thoughts and behaviors, and to let go of them. Practical spirituality helps you to learn how to accept your life and your emotions for what they are, rather than wishing things were different. (You'll also explore a more active approach to this when you learn how to manage stress through refocusing stress producing thoughts in chapter 6.)

For example, Jane, a fifty-year-old cancer survivor, felt as if cancer had bored a hole in her life. This hole began to feel especially deep after her children moved out of the house. She felt that she needed something more in her life, but wasn't a religious person in a traditional sense. Although she attended support groups, she still felt something was missing.

So Jane looked into practical spirituality. She began meditating, reframing her negative thoughts, and trying to reign her thoughts in to focus only on the present moment. She stopped worrying about the future and regretting the past. She also worked hard to forgive. Jane told me that she found the meditation particularly helpful, because it allows her to train her mind to stay focused on the present.

After practicing this form of spirituality for some time, Jane began to feel calmer and more peaceful. These strategies have helped her figure out what is really important to her at this point in her life—such as her children and their future, and her relationship with her husband and other close members of her family.

In the following pages, you'll find a number of components of practical spirituality to try. If this approach sounds like it might be helpful and simple to use, I strongly encourage you to explore this topic further.

> ### *Survivor Stat*
>
> RESEARCH SUGGESTS that many cancer survivors are changed by their experience, often for years after treatment has ended. Stressful and traumatic life events such as cancer can have a strong positive impact on individuals, causing them to "make meaning" out of their struggle. Studies show that after cancer treatment, many survivors experience a better appreciation of life and improved relationships with friends and families.

Thought Watching

Sit down in a quiet place. Close your eyes. Take a few deep breaths to relax and turn your awareness inward. Try to watch your mind as if you are a casual observer.

Don't judge or try to manipulate your thoughts. Just notice them. As your thoughts pass through your mind like clouds, try to notice which ones dwell in the future. These thoughts tend to start with the phase, "What if . . . ?" Also, try to notice which thoughts dwell on past events. These thoughts tend to start with the phrase, "If only . . ."

Also, notice how these thoughts tend to make you feel. If any thought makes you feel strongly—good or bad—write it down. Do this once a day for a week, and then look over your thought journal and see if there is a pattern to your thoughts and feelings.

Then, do the same exercise again, every day for a second week. During this second round, see if you can let the thoughts go. As they pass through your mind, notice whether they dwell in the past or future. Congratulate yourself for becoming aware of them, and then let them drift out of your mind, just as if they were clouds gently blowing their way across the sky.

Basic Meditation

Yogis believe that meditation can help you to organize your mind. As you meditate—and therefore focus your thoughts—you are able to get in touch with what they call "the true self." Similar to the Christian description of a "soul," the true self is always there, but never changes. Getting in touch with it can help you to keep your focus on what's most important, and ignore the usual frustrating aspects of life that maybe are not as important as you initially thought.

To slow down and focus your mind, try this simple meditation.

1. Sit or lie in a comfortable position.
2. Close your eyes and take several deep, relaxing breaths. Each time you exhale, feel your body grow heavier and more relaxed. Visualize the tension leaving your body with each breath.
3. Once you are relaxed, silently hear the sound "soooo" as you inhale. As you exhale, mentally say the sound "hummm" to yourself.
4. Try to keep your focus on these sounds. Your mind will wander. That's normal. Whenever you catch stray thoughts running through your mind, just gently bring your focus back to the sounds "so" and "hum."

At first, you might only be able to focus on these sounds for a minute. Over time, you might deepen your practice to twenty minutes.

Zen Meditation

This form of meditation encourages you to focus on the present moment. No matter what you are doing, you immerse all of your senses on the task at hand. Let's say you are washing the dishes. Rather than rushing through the task, trying to finish the mundane task as fast as you can, do the following:

1. Notice the temperature of the water over your hands.
2. Listen to the sounds of the water as it rushes into the sink.
3. Smell the scent of dishwashing liquid.
4. Watch the bubbles of soap as you scrub the plates. See the water wash both the bubbles and the grime away. Try to notice every visual detail.

As you immerse yourself in the present, your anxiety about the future and your regret about the past melt away. The more often you try to do this, the less often you will find yourself worrying about upcoming tests, fretting about problems at work, or feeling remorseful over your lot in life.

Loving Kindness Meditation

This type of meditation can help you shed pent-up anger, guilt, and other negative emotions. It can also help you to forgive others and shed old resentments. Do the following:

1. Sit or lie in a comfortable position.
2. Close your eyes and take several deep, relaxing breaths. Each time you exhale, feel your body grow heavier and more relaxed. Visualize the tension leaving your body with each breath.
3. One you feel relaxed, you'll bring the image of three people to mind: one of yourself, one of a loved one, and one of someone who makes you feel anger or some other negative emotion.
4. One by one, bring the images of these people to mind, starting first with yourself.
5. Visualize each person in front of you. If need be, forgive this person and visualize yourself sending warm, bright, loving-kindness energy from your heart to theirs. See this person light up with your gift.
6. Hold this image in your mind for a few moments and then release the image of this person from your mind. Repeat for all three images.

Although this exercise may seem challenging at first, have faith and persevere. You'll be surprised at just how effectively it can help you to shed old resentments.

SUPPORT GROUPS

I'VE SEEN BOTH sides of the coin when it comes to support groups. Before my diagnosis, I used to run support groups for breast cancer survivors. After my diagnosis, I found myself seated as a participant in a support group for brain cancer survivors. These experiences have taught me something that may at first seem quite controversial: support groups are not for everyone!

Although support groups can be very helpful for some survivors, others may find them a waste of time, and still others may find that these groups remind them of cancer and keep them mired in the past. If the latter describes you, know that there are lots of ways to get the support you want and need. Support groups provide just one avenue toward your goal. So don't feel bad if you tried one for a while but decided not go back, or if you've always felt you should try one but just don't seem to get around to doing it. You may have very real reasons for not getting involved.

Before you give up on support groups entirely, however, consider whether you gave the support group a real chance. Perhaps a different type of support group could help you more than the one you tried. You might prefer a group with a different mix of survivors, for example, or with a different moderator. You may feel more comfortable in a smaller group or in a larger group.

I suggest this because support groups can be very helpful, especially if you find a good one that meets your personal needs. In the beginning of your survivorship journey, these groups can provide useful information that you can use to improve your health, health care, and mood. For those so inclined, these groups can also provide a safe place for you to talk out some of the fears and anxieties that you don't feel comfortable sharing with family and friends. Those dark fears of recurrences, memories of your response to your diagnosis or your treatments, and the dread you may have about death are all fair game at a support group. You need not worry about bringing down the other members.

When choosing a support group, consider carefully who is leading the discussion. There are many types of groups. Some are led by professionals, others by lay counselors or lay people who want to help, and still others led by cancer survivors. Some focus on solving problems whereas others have little focus at all. Survivors simply talk about whatever comes to mind. Ideally, you want a moderator who can keep the group focused on solving problems rather than simply wallowing in problems, one who can offer helpful advice in a pinch as well as encourage others in the group to share their helpful experiences, encouraging the group to solve problems together. (Consult Appendix A for a listing of support group resources).

In a recent review of more than 1,400 cancer survivors, my research group found that treatments that taught survivors specific strategies, such as problem solving or stress-reduction tactics, had a greater positive effect on depression, anxiety, and quality of life over three months than groups that just provided general knowledge about cancer and survivorship. When sampling groups and finding one to call home, consider the following questions carefully:

- Does someone keep things rolling along and focused on useful views and approaches to problems, or does the group become a gripe session about doctors and symptoms? In other words, does the group focus on productive conversation or does it turn into—as my son would say—a pity fest?
- Does the moderator allow one or two people to dominate the group? If so, this will prevent you from expressing your views and getting helpful feedback.
- Do group members come from all stages of survivorship (including newly diagnosed, currently involved in their major treatment, those who are further along and had major treatment years ago, relatives who have lost loved ones to cancer)? The more varied the group, the broader the discussion.
- Similarly, does the group include survivors who have battled all types of cancer or does it center mainly on just one type of cancer?
- Why do you attend the group? Does it give you what you want and need? Does it fill an emotional void?

Once you begin going to a group on a regular basis, consider carefully the advice you get from the other survivors in the group. Although other survivors can be very helpful and encouraging, they are not doctors. It's easy to get caught up in the hope that a treatment that worked for one survivor will also work for you. Remember that every person and every situation is different. Investigate information you receive from a support group with the same rigor as you would from a news report. Do your Internet and medical database search. Read the research and consult your doctor.

I am not suggesting that the advice you hear at a support group is all a bunch of hogwash. Not at all. I'm only recommending that you treat the advice and information you hear, including the guidance in this book, with a sense of realistic optimism.

GIVING BACK

MANY CANCER SURVIVORS appreciate life much more after cancer than they did before. This appreciation often translates into a need to give back to the community and make the world a better place.

Cancer survivorship provides some time to step back and consider things you have not done in the past. You can travel or spend more time with family and friends. You can also explore the idea of spending some time

How Support Groups Can Help

BELOW YOU'LL FIND a letter that a support-group member wrote. It illustrates the degree of support, good will, and positive attitude that can emanate from survivors who are members of such groups.

To all Survivors and friends:

Another month has passed and hopefully another month of miracles for each of us. I know I feel personally blessed to have shared a part of your lives (OK, maybe not the best part, BUT certainly a critical part), and have learned from each of you about the strength and resolve of the human spirit.

Please plan to attend to help yourselves, but also to help others. Your journey through this brain tumor morass will certainly be of interest to all of us, but could prove crucial to one similarly situated to see the light in your eyes, the spring in your step, and your positive attitude about the "Long and Winding Road" of survivorship.

As Always: Every first Thursday of each month.

with others that may need your help. This often can help you feel more useful. By doing something for others who are in need of your support, you can feel better about your survival. Many cancer survivors volunteer with cancer organizations. Whether they work for survivor organizations or for cancer-specific groups, almost all of these individuals will tell you that it feels good to give back to others in need. Of course, it does not have to be a cancer group. Any type of altruistic activity often helps those who get involved, as well as the recipients.

Consider the following ways to give back to the community, in ways directly related to cancer or not:

- Help raise money for cancer research.
- Sign up, form a team, and train for a race (such as the Race for the Cure series) that raises money for cancer research or to help cancer patients.

- Volunteer for social service organizations, such as the American Cancer Society or a non–cancer related organization such as the American Heart Association, your local parent-teacher organization, food bank, or religious community.
- Join an online network sponsored by the American Cancer Society.
- Ask a local hospital, long-term care facility, or rehabilitation facility how you can volunteer to help others who are battling cancer.
- Volunteer to lead a cancer support group.
- Volunteer to serve as a patient navigator for someone who is battling cancer.
- Donate money to a charitable cause.
- Volunteer at a summer camp for children with cancer or other types of health conditions.

Need other ideas? Try Network for Good (www.networkforgood) or contact your local township office.

In the end, giving your support *to* others is just as important as getting support *from* others. I think you will find, as I have, that the more you give of yourself, the more you receive in return. As you immerse yourself in such volunteer efforts, you'll be rewarded not only with a greater sense of meaning and purpose, but also with a strong, supportive community of other cancer survivors. The more races you run, support groups you facilitate, or patients you visit in the hospital, the more people you know and feel close with. This type of strong, large, tightly woven community is perhaps the most important type of support of all. So give and give freely. Help others as you help yourself.

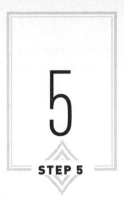

STEP 5

Find the Courage to Change

"**WHY DID I** get cancer?" It's easy to get caught up trying to find an answer to this question. When I was diagnosed with a brain tumor, for example, of course I wanted to know why. I read scientific studies about the causes of brain tumors, consulted with many doctors and scientists in this country and around the world, and spent a lot of time pondering whether my past habits of using a cell phone and eating (or not eating) certain foods were to blame. I eventually discovered that the ventilation system in the building where I work had spread toxic chemicals into the air. Other employees had developed brain, stomach, and other types of cancer. I thought, "This is it. This is what caused my cancer!"

Over a year and a half, I spent countless hours trying to document the link between the chemical exposures at work and cancer. I got nowhere. After all, cancer is caused by many factors, not just one. I couldn't prove anything. My employer had already installed a new ventilation system in my building. I realized my search was only doing one thing: wasting time and energy that I could have put toward recovering from my treatments, preventing a recurrence, and improving my health and the quality of my life.

Indeed, as I learned, at some point after our diagnoses, we survivors must stop living in the past and begin to look forward to the future. To do so, we must spend the time and energy needed to improve our health and quality of life. It not only will help prevent a recurrence, but also will help improve your energy, and mental and physical functioning. Too often, however, cancer survivors don't do this, and the reasons are varied.

Many of us easily get caught up in the past. That's one reason. Another: the cancer and its treatments can sometimes make it difficult to live health-fully. Fatigue makes exercise challenging. You may have lost your appetite for certain foods or actually increased your eating to accommodate an increase in appetite because of the medication you needed to take during treatment. Lingering memory or organizational problems may cause undue stress. You've probably been told that you must learn to live with a new sense of what is "normal," that your life will never be the same as it was before cancer. While this is true, it doesn't give you an excuse to give up. You can get healthy. You can learn to enjoy life again. You can lose weight, exercise, and eat right. The advice in this chapter will help you to make your health and daily functioning as close to "normal" as possible.

Some cancer survivors—myself included—try to reason their way out of exercising and improving their lifestyle with the following: "Why bother? I've already been diagnosed with a deadly illness. What other health prob-lems could I possibly get?" Unfortunately the answer to that question is, "anything and everything." Your odds of developing another serious ill-ness, such as heart disease or diabetes, are the same or greater than that of the nonsurvivor. Recent studies conclude that a cancer diagnosis does not immunize you against other diseases!

To illustrate this point, I'd like to tell you the story of a young accoun-tant I once knew, named Barbara. She had survived breast cancer. She had survived the worst, therefore, nothing else could happen, she told me. She had two kids, a good marriage, and was working to become a partner at her firm. Due to her demanding work and parenting life, she felt she couldn't take time for her own needs. Over time, she gained weight, ate poorly, did not exercise, and, consequently, developed diabetes. At age forty-five, she had a stroke, which made it even more of a challenge to keep up with work and her two children, ages thirteen and eight. Somehow, she never saw it coming.

Don't follow in Barbara's footsteps! Make a promise to yourself right now that you will read the rest of this chapter and, based on what you learn, make one change in your life *today* that will improve your health and quality of life. That's not a lot. I'm not suggesting you do everything at once. Tomorrow, you don't need to jump out of bed and start exercising, quit smoking, begin eating more fruits and vegetables, hire a personal trainer, lose weight, and reduce the amount of fat in your diet. No, I'm just suggesting you make one change. Just one. You owe it to yourself. You've survived cancer after all. You need to stay healthy!

GETTING READY FOR CHANGE

EXERCISING, EATING RIGHT, maintaining a normal weight, and not smoking are important for all people, not just cancer survivors. Yet, they may be even more important for survivors, as these healthful habits might prevent a recurrence, or, more likely, another deadly disease such as heart disease or diabetes. These habits can also help alleviate fatigue and other treatment-induced symptoms.

Yet, those treatment-induced symptoms make it tougher for us to adopt and maintain the very habits that will help us feel better. According to an American Cancer Society survey, only 47 percent of survivors improved their dietary habits after their diagnosis, only 47 percent of smokers quit, and a startling 30 percent exercised *less*.

To help increase your success at adopting and maintaining healthful habits, take the following self-assessment, Can I Change? It will give you a realistic view of how willing you are to make a change—any change—in your life. All too often, we say that we want to lose weight, start an exercise program, change our diet, or drink less alcohol, but we don't really mean it. Yes, we want to change, but we don't want to invest the time and energy needed to make the change happen.

The self-assessment below is intended to help you better understand your motivations to change, as well as make you aware of how difficult some areas are to change. You need to be aware that the ability to change may become influenced by newer treatments that are developed all the time. For example, quitting smoking has become a little easier for some with the development of the nicotine patch, just as dieting has become a little easier with more variety in the available dietetic foods. With this in mind, this self-assessment will help you connect those two important factors, helping you to see what's really holding you back from making true, lasting change in your life. There are few structured ways for you to really think this through, so I thought this quiz would be very informative for you. Take it. I think you'll find the results both surprising and informative. Most important, what you learn from this self-assessment will help you to better structure your program for change, increasing your chances of success.

Before taking the quiz, identify the one change you wish to make (starting an exercise program, eating a healthier diet, lowering your cholesterol or blood sugar, controlling your depression, losing weight, or stopping smoking). With that change in mind, use the self-assessment to get an idea of just how challenging it will be for you to make this change. Then,

Can I Change?

◈

THIS SELF-ASSESSMENT WILL help you to determine your chances of changing a lifestyle behavior (such as starting an exercise program) based on the odds (found in research on people who actually attempted to make those lifestyle changes), your past history of trying to change these habits, and your current feelings about change.

CAN I CHANGE?

BEHAVIOR YOU WANT TO CHANGE	THE ODDS—BASED ON RESEARCH—THAT YOU CAN SUCCESSFULLY MAKE THIS LIFESTYLE CHANGE	CIRCLE ONE NUMBER BELOW THAT CORRESPONDS TO ONE CHANGE YOU WISH TO MAKE
Stop Smoking	9%	.09
Lose Weight	5%	.05
Lift Depression	70%	.7
Exercise	35%	.35
Stop Drinking Alcohol	10%	.1
Lower Cholesterol Through Diet	50%	.5
(A) Write the number you circled here:		

STAGE OF CHANGE YOU ARE NOW IN	WHAT IT MEANS	CIRCLE ONE NUMBER BELOW THAT BEST DESCRIBES HOW YOU FEEL ABOUT MAKING THIS CHANGE
You haven't thought about changing until you took this quiz, and even now, it's not really on your radar.	You're unlikely to change.	1
You realize you need to change and you're thinking about doing so, but you have not formulated a plan.	You might change.	2
You know that you need to do something and you have a plan to get it done.	You're likely to change.	3
	(B) Write the number you circled here:	

YOUR TRACK RECORD		CIRCLE THE NUMBER THAT BEST DESCRIBES YOUR TRACK RECORD OF CHANGING THIS BEHAVIOR IN THE PAST.
You've never changed this behavior in the past.		1
You've changed before, but relapsed within one month.		2

YOUR TRACK RECORD	CIRCLE THE NUMBER THAT BEST DESCRIBES YOUR TRACK RECORD OF CHANGING THIS BEHAVIOR IN THE PAST.
You've changed before, but relapsed in six months.	3
You've changed before, but relapsed within one year.	4
You've changed before, but relapsed only after you kept the change going for more than a year.	5
	(C) Write the number you circled here:
Chance of Success in Changing Behavior	Add up the numbers you wrote down for A, B, and C

* Developed from and used with permission from R. E. Feinstein and M. S. Feinstein. "Psychotherapy for Health and Lifestyle Change." *Journal of Clinical Psychology.* 57, no. 11 (2001):1263–75

What Your Score Means: The higher your total for A + B + C, the greater your chances of successfully changing this behavior.

use the advice throughout this chapter to increase your chances of making successful and lasting lifestyle changes.

Once you determine your score, then read this paragraph, because you'll probably need this little pep talk. You might be wondering about the chances of you losing weight given that only 5 percent of us really manage to do it successfully. That is what this exercise is all about—showing you what you are really up against. Try not to get discouraged and mutter, "Well, why even bother changing? There's no way I can lose what I need to!" Rather, use the information to your advantage, as a catalyst for change. So, for example, let's say your score is pretty low. What can you do? Rather than give up, spend more time thinking about strategies that can increase the chances that your effort will work.

How to Improve Your Success

If you have many lifestyle changes you'd like to make, use the quiz to help prioritize which change to tackle first. For example, let's say you'd like to stop smoking and to lose weight. You take the quiz twice, once for each goal. For smoking, (0.09), you realize you need to do it but have not formulated a plan (2), and you have stopped smoking before, only to relapse within six months (4). Your total comes to 6.09. For weight loss (0.5), you really have not thought about it much (1) and you never have tried to lose weight in the past (1). Your total is 2.5. The higher the score the more likely you can change the habit.

Based on the two results, you can see that, although both are important for your health, it will be easier for you to stop smoking than to lose weight. It does not mean that smoking cessation will be easy. It will just be easier than losing weight. So try giving up the smokes first, and then losing weight second.

In addition to helping you to prioritize your goals, the quiz can help you to see just how challenging your lifestyle change will become. The range of scores from the self-assessment range from a low of 2.09 to a high of 8.7. If you score in the low range, let's say below 5, for some habit you really need to change, you should expect that you are very likely to face a bumpy road ahead. This doesn't mean you will for sure or that you should give up. Rather, it means you need to take some proactive steps to prepare for your program. For example, if your goal is to begin an exercise program, you might need to work with a fitness partner or fitness guide. If weight loss is your goal, consider enrolling in a more structured weight-control program, such as Weight Watchers, to really get this going and to increase your success. Here are some ways to improve your score—and, therefore, your chances of success—in the three areas of that the self-assessment covers:

Behavior you wish or need to change: Focus on making just one change at a time. For example, start an exercise program. Once that's underway, then improve your diet. Once you've made that change, then quit smoking. Don't do it all at once.

Your stage of change: To be successful, you must really see the importance of changing. To do so, think about the positive reasons for taking on this change, along with the negative aspects of doing nothing. Consult Weighing Your Pros and Cons, page 117, for help. Most health professionals consider cancer survivors to be more open to change after cancer; use that to your advantage and focus on the positive reasons you need to change. But be realistic: remember, even the American Cancer Society has shown that only about half of cancer survivors really change their health habits once they have cancer.

Your track record: If you have tried to change before but failed, it doesn't mean you'll fail this time around. In fact, research done on smokers and dieters shows that many people fail at lifestyle changes many times before they succeed. So, don't give up! Use your past attempts at change to your advantage. For help in doing just that, consult Improving Your track Record on page 118.

GET MOVING

OF ALL THE changes you can make to improve your health, well-being, and outlook on life, exercise is perhaps the most important—and simultaneously most challenging change to tackle.

First, let's take a look at why *all* cancer survivors need exercise. Many doctors like to joke that if they could compact all of the benefits of exercise and put them into a pill, they'd be millionaires. In addition to strengthening your muscles, regular exercise:

- *Strengthens your bones:* This is particularly important for young women survivors who were thrust into early menopause either due to a hysterectomy or chemotherapy-induced ovarian damage. The resulting lack

Weighing Your Pros and Cons

IN THE SPACE provided below, write down all the positive consequences of changing (such as a longer life, more energy, and better mood) as well as the negative consequences of not changing (such as the money you spend on cigarettes.)

If I change, how will it positively impact the following aspects of my life:

Health: _____

_____

Relationships: _____

_____

Mood: _____

_____

Energy level: _____

_____

Employment: _____

_____

Financial status: _____

_____

If I don't change, how will my current lifestyle affect the following:

Health: _____

_____

Relationships: _____

_____

Mood: _____

_____

Energy level: _____

_____

Employment: _____

_____

Financial status: _____

_____

Improving Your Track Record

THINK BACK TO your past attempts to change. What you did well and what you could improve? What tripped you up and why? How can you do it differently this time to circumvent such obstacles? To improve your chances of success this time around, consider the following tactics:

- Increase your support by asking your spouse or friend to make the change with you.
- Keep tabs on your progress. For exercise, write the workouts you intend to complete on a calendar and then check them off as you complete them. For nutrition, keep a food log, writing down what you eat. At the end of each day, look it over and brainstorm ways to do better. For smoking, put a star on your calendar every time you get through a usual smoking period smoke-free.

of estrogen can allow your bones to weaken. However, regular weight-bearing exercise, such as walking and weight lifting, can encourage your bones to hold onto calcium and other minerals.

- *Condition your body:* Cancer treatment takes a toll on the body. Chemotherapy in particular—along with the assorted medications you may have taken to counteract common side effects—tends to cause either weight gain and weight loss. During your treatments, you may have felt too sick to move. All of that bedrest and sitting have caused your muscles and heart to weaken. The only way to strengthen them: exercise.
- *Boosts energy levels:* Recent research shows that physical exercise is the only drug-free way to combat the fatigue so many of us battle after cancer treatment. Physical exercise leads to an increase in functional capacity, requiring less effort from you to perform activities.
- *Improves mood:* As you'll learn in chapter 6, cancer treatment can also change your brain chemistry, making you more prone to depression. Many studies show that aerobic exercise helps lift depression, often as effectively as medication. Just as important if you reduce your exercise activity, or worse yet, stop completely, it can cause depression. In one study completed on twenty-four depressed breast cancer survivors, ten weeks of aerobic exercise (four days a week, thirty to forty minutes per

session) reduced depression and anxiety significantly over a control group that did not exercise.

That's the positive, optimistic view. Now, let's get realistic. Let's take a look at why you might find exercise challenging so you can take the steps necessary to overcome those challenges to lifestyle change. First, and most important, you probably are in a deconditioned state. Even if you were fit before your cancer treatments, you might find the simplest tasks—such as climbing a flight of stairs—challenging. Also, your treatments may have caused some damage in various parts of your body, making certain types of exercise more difficult. For example, if you had surgery, scar tissue may rule out or require you to be more careful with certain weight lifting or stretching movements.

The best way to deal with those challenges? Set conservative goals. You probably will not reach all your goals at once nor will you achieve the fitness level of someone like Lance Armstrong. You don't have to in order to improve your general physical health, well-being, and quality of life. Each week, make it your goal to do a little more than you did the week before. If you currently do no exercise, start with just ten minutes. If you usually take a short morning walk with the dog, add another short walk in the evening. Eventually, you want to work up to thirty to forty-five minutes of daily activity most days of the week. (Consult your physician for advice about the best exercise program for your particular situation).

> ### *Survivor Stat*
>
> ADULT CANCER survivors who exercise three times per week report a significantly higher quality of life than survivors who do not exercise or who exercise less often.

The American College of Sports Medicine recommends the following:

- Exercise 3 to 5 days each week.
- Warm up for 5 to 10 minutes before aerobic activity.
- Maintain your exercise intensity for 30 to 45 minutes.
- Gradually decrease the intensity of your workout, then stretch to cool down during the last 5 to 10 minutes.
- If weight loss is major goal, participate in aerobic activity at least 30 minutes for 5 days each week.

For more information about exercise, go to the ACSM Web site (www .acsm.org). There, you will find a simple tool to help you monitor your heart rate, along with recommendations on how to purchase exercise equipment and find personal trainers. Of course, while it may help, you do not need to purchase equipment or hire a personal trainer to improve your level of fitness.

Here are some additional tips for starting—and maintaining—an exercise program.

Go to a gym. Research shows that group fitness programs increase participation and results over home-based programs. The other participants in the class—who will miss you if you don't show up—will motivate you to stick with your routine.

Get a workout buddy. Walk with a friend, spouse, or neighbor. Meet someone at the gym for a workout. This buddy will help hold you to your schedule, helping to motivate you to put on your sneakers when you'd rather take a nap on the couch. You may find it especially helpful to exercise with another cancer survivor.

Sign up for a few sessions with a personal trainer. In addition to helping you to find the best weight-lifting exercises and stretches for you, this person will help make you accountable to your program. More important, your trainer can help to design a program for you to overcome certain exercise challenges, such as surgical pain. You can ask for this assistance at most gyms. Many hospitals have people on staff who will work with you to set up an exercise program. You can also see a physical therapist or exercise physiologist.

Keep track of your workouts. On a calendar, day planner, or even an ordinary sheet of paper you keep taped to the fridge, write down the date, time, intensity (example: treadmill at level 4), and duration (example: 30 minutes) of your exercise sessions. Keep track of amount of weight you lift, and your heart rate during cardiovascular exercise. This type of record keeping can help you see your results more easily. For example, as you increase the intensity and or duration of your exercise plan, your heart rate will increase at first, but over time it will level out, indicating that your heart is actually tolerating more physical activity and that your endurance is improving.

Keep a regular schedule. Exercise at the same time every day. Regularity will make it feel like a scheduled task to be completed.

Define Your Roadblocks to Exercise

THIS QUIZ WILL help you to identify ways to increase your physical activity. Circle Yes or No for each of the following statements:

1. I like to exercise.	Yes	No
2. My friends exercise, so I think I should.	Yes	No
3. I always do what I plan to do.	Yes	No
4. Exercise is difficult for me.	Yes	No
5. I exercise with friends.	Yes	No
6. Exercise is good for me.	Yes	No
7. I have set a goal for exercise.	Yes	No
8. My doctor thinks I should exercise.	Yes	No
9. If I wanted to, I could exercise regularly.	Yes	No
10. I plan to exercise regularly every week.	Yes	No
11. I can exercise any time of the day I want.	Yes	No
12. I am confident I can exercise.	Yes	No

Questions 1, 4, and 6 tell you about your **attitude** toward exercise.

Questions 3, 7, and 10 tell you about your **intention** to follow through on your exercise plan.

Questions 9, 11, and 12 tell you about your **confidence** in your ability to actually do the exercise (e.g., lift the weights) that you have planned.

Questions 2, 5, and 8 tell you how much **others influence** your decision to exercise.

Ideally, you want to answer yes to all of the questions. Define the area (attitude, intentions, confidence, and others' influence) where you have the fewest yes responses. Consult the area that needs attention (attitude, intentions, confidence) in the pages that follow for advice on how to improve your score—and remove your roadblocks to exercising.

Invest in appropriate exercise clothing or accessories. The more comfortable you feel while exercising, the more you'll feel like exercising. Invest in a good, comfortable pair of shoes designed for the activity you plan to do. In other words, if you will be walking, get walking shoes. If you'll be running, get running shoes. If you'll be doing aerobics and other types of classes, get cross-trainers or aerobic-style shoes. Visit a sports specific shoe store to be properly fitted. Some of these stores employ experts in shoe fitting. These folks can help ensure that the shoe you buy works best for your foot and activity type.

In addition to shoes, you'll also need comfortable clothing. Also, consider investing in a CD player or MP3 player, as listening to your favorite music will make walking or running more interesting.

When you're tired, just do ten minutes. When you're tempted to skip your exercise routine because you feel too tired or too hurried, commit yourself to just ten minutes. Put on your walking shoes and just do it. If after ten minutes you still feel tired, then go home and rest! Chances are, however, that, once you rev up your heart rate, you'll start to feel good and want to keep walking!

Removing your Roadblocks

Take the quiz on page 121 to define precisely what's stopping you from starting or maintaining an exercise program. Then, with your results in hand, use the following strategies to remove your roadblocks to exercise for each area defined by the quiz.

Intentions: Even though we all *want* to change, sometimes we need a little nudge to actually create the plan that will translate our desire to change into results. Make sure your plan is something you are serious about being able to accomplish. If not, think about which parts you are unsure about, and then modify them to help you reach your intended goal. You may have several smaller plans that come together to reach the larger goal. As they say, Rome was not built in a day, and it usually takes a couple of weeks, or longer, to change a behavior.

To come up with your plan, consult your doctor, a therapist or the trainers at your local gym. Start at your own pace though and make your plan something that is easy for you to put into place. For example, you could try walking around the track at your local high school, finding an exercise partner and committing to exercise three times a week, or joining the local YMCA or other fitness center. You just want to get moving.

Use the following to guide your planning efforts.

Activity I will do: _____

What equipment, if any, I will use: _____

_____

How often I will exercise: _____

Who will help keep me motivated: _____

What I hope to gain from exercising:_____

_____

How I will keep my attitude positive about exercising: _____

_____

_____

Date I will start: _____

How I will know when I've reached my goal (even my shorter term goals):

_____

_____

_____

If I stop exercising and become frustrated, what can I do? ___

_____

Call a friend? Who? _____

What will I reward myself with for sticking to the plan and achieving the goal?

_____

_____

_____

Attitude: A good attitude about exercising makes you more likely to follow through on your plan. Conversely, exercise can also improve your attitude! More physical activity can have a positive effect on your emotional as well as physical well-being. You may feel less tired once you are exercising. Being aware of the payoff will keep you focused on the long run. Also, work on changing your attitude or beliefs about activity or exercise. Answer the question, "how is this really going to help me?" You have to believe in the outcome to stick to your plan.

Confidence: When you are confident in your abilities, you feel that you can be physically active, know how equipment works for your choice of activity, or know what you really need to do to get the most out of your exercise time. For example, you can operate a rowing machine or treadmill comfortably, or know what level your heart rate needs to get to and how much time you need for it to recover to a pre-exercise level. To improve your confidence, sign up for a few sessions with a personal trainer, physical therapist, or another professional who can help you create a program specific to your needs.

Others' influence: If a doctor recommends that you exercise, you are more likely to exercise. Even though it may seem as though they are pestering you, your friends' or spouses' repeated suggestions to exercise can eventually help convince you to exercise. For example, will you do it just to please your wife? To not be afraid the next time you go to a doctor's appointment and have to admit that you have not followed his or her advice? Regardless of who is pressuring you do it, the fact is that you know exercise is good for you and that person is looking out for your own best interests, so get out there and get moving.

Track Your Progress

Once you get started, you may find that keeping track of your progress may help you see how you are doing. For example, track the number of minutes that you exercise (in five-minute increments) on a graph like the one below. Here is an example for you:

TRACK YOUR PROGRESS							
Place an *x* in the box under each day to show how many minutes you have exercised each day. Then connect the *x* marks to see the trend.							
MINUTES	**SUN**	**MON**	**TUES**	**WED**	**THUR**	**FRI**	**SAT**
60							
55							
50							
45							
40							
35					x	x	
30							
25		x					x
20				x			
15							
10	x						
5			x				

Here is a blank form for you to use. You may want to make several copies, so you can track yourself over the long run. Doing so will not only keep you interested in your program, but you can use it to show your doctor what you have been doing. Don't forget to reward yourself after reaching a goal of keeping up your exercise. Try treating yourself to a new outfit if the goal is to exercise and lose weight. Or give yourself a new CD for your CD player if you are using that to help you exercise. Good luck!

TRACK YOUR PROGRESS							
Place an *x* in the box under each day to show how many minutes you have exercised each day. Then connect the *x* marks to see the trend.							
MINUTES	SUN	MON	TUES	WED	THUR	FRI	SAT
60							
55							
50							
45							
40							
35							
30							
25							
20							
15							
10							
5							

IMPROVE YOUR DIET

COUNTLESS STUDIES SHOW that food truly is medicine. The pigments in orange, red, green, yellow, and other brightly colored vegetables—what scientists collectively call phytochemicals—may prevent a host of diseases, including cancer and heart disease. At the very least, they can help keep us generally healthy. A healthful diet can help improve energy levels and strength, keep your weight in check, improve immunity, and speed healing.

Unfortunately, most of us don't eat enough of these power foods. For example, one study of breast cancer survivors determined that survivors tended to eat too few grains, vegetables, fruits, milk, and meat, and too much overall fat, saturated fat, cholesterol, and sodium. Sodium scores were particularly high. These survivors also tended to eat the same foods day after day rather than the wide variety of foods that nutrition experts recommend.

Why might survivors eat so poorly? The answer varies from person to person. For some survivors, lingering side effects from treatments may be at fault. Cancer and cancer treatments can alter your body's ability to tolerate certain foods, reduce your appetite, and change your sense of taste or smell. You simply may find that you can't stomach certain foods. As with most challenges, you can overcome this, and you don't have to force yourself to eat something you hate! There are many, many different types of healthful foods on the planet. Adopt a sense of adventure. During each trip to the grocery store, put a new fruit, vegetable, whole grain, or legume in the cart and try it. Eventually, you'll find an assortment of healthful foods that you like to eat.

Also, consider meeting with a registered dietitian who specializes in cancer and cancer survival. These professionals can not only help you craft a diet that helps you eat more nutritiously—no matter the posttreatment changes to your taste buds—but also one that includes phytochemicals and other nutrients that the body can use to detoxify carcinogens and inhibit tumor-producing genes.

To improve your diet, do the following:

- Eat five to seven servings of fruits and vegetables (make sure some of these servings include citrus, dark leafy greens, cruciferous vegetables such as broccoli, and deep yellow veggies) every day.
- Consume numerous servings of whole-grain foods every day. Replace refined grains, such as white bread and white rice, with whole-grain versions, such as brown rice and whole wheat bread.
- Replace products high in saturated fats (butter) and trans fats (margarine and many processed foods) with foods high in monounsaturated fats such as olive oil. Other healthful fat sources include nuts, avocados, olives, and natural peanut butter.
- Whenever possible, choose trans fat–free versions of such processed foods as breakfast cereal, snack crackers, and bread. Reduce the amount of saturated fat in your diet by using fat-free or reduced-fat dairy and meat products, such as skim milk, ground sirloin, and skinless turkey breast.

- Eat coldwater fatty fish such as salmon, or a flax product such as flaxseed oil, flax seeds, or flax meal twice a week.
- Drink alcohol only occasionally, holding yourself to one or fewer alcoholic drinks a day. Although moderate drinking may reduce risk for heart disease, it can raise risk for breast cancer.
- Do not eat salt-cured, smoked, or pickled foods, for the same reason.

To get a handle on your diet and gain the motivation you need to change it, keep a food diary. Each day, write down what you eat. At the end of the day, add up your fruit and vegetable servings. Also, look at your grain products. Could you have chosen a whole-grain version instead? Even if you think you eat healthfully, you may be surprised by your results.

For more nutritional information, go to the American Cancer Society (www.cancer.org) or the U.S. Department of Health and Human Services Web sites (www.hhs.gov).

MANAGE YOUR WEIGHT

MANY CANCER SURVIVORS find themselves heavier after treatment for cancer. As many of us can attest to, some of the medications used to control inflammation or swelling (such as steroid drugs) affect appetite. These medications often trigger overeating. Coupled with the inactivity that's common after surgery and other treatments, many survivors find themselves much heavier than before their diagnoses. Also, if you are a breast, ovarian, cervical, or uterine cancer survivor, your treatments may have thrust you into early menopause. Among other things, your reduced levels of estrogen will cause you to lose muscle mass at a faster rate, slow your metabolism, and encourage weight gain in your abdomen.

I know this struggle well. I gained as much as twenty pounds by the time I finished all my major treatments for cancer. Some this excess weight stemmed from the steroids I took, which increased my appetite to a level I never thought was possible. I also was less active during this time, preferring to sit around rather than get out and walk. This combination of increased eating and less activity was a double whammy.

Months and years passed, and while my activity level increased (it never got up to where it was before the cancer), it did not compensate for my eating. Although I was not gaining weight, I was not losing it, either. I knew that I really needed to do something (plus, my doctor and my wife mentioned my need to do something quite regularly!), but still I was eating too much and not exercising enough. So I signed up for a service that helps people control how much they eat by providing tasty healthy foods . . . real food, yet portion and calorie controlled. (You can replicate the same type of program by purchasing prepared low-calorie meals at the grocery store or following low-calorie recipes.) My wife ate these meals as well, so we were losing weight together, which helped keep me motivated. I have not felt this energetic in so long that it actually feels strange to me! We have stopped the program, but my portions are smaller and I am now committed to losing another ten pounds. This way I will be back to what I weighed before the cancer.

Years ago I had conducted research for a weight loss company and reported on barriers to successful weight loss. I uncovered many factors that influenced whether people stuck with a weight loss program and actually lost weight. I created a Weight Loss Profile that clients could use to become more aware of their potential barriers to successful weight loss. There were a number of weight loss barriers that we documented. Two of them were:

- *Impatience:* Many people want to lose weight fast yet, to keep the weight off, you must become comfortable with slow, steady weight loss. Studies show that people who keep weight off long term lost weight at a rate of just one to two pounds a week. This slower-paced weight loss helps preserve muscle mass and your metabolic rate. When you lose weight too quickly, your body burns muscle protein—as well as fat—for fuel. Not only does this make you tired and weaker, it also slows your metabolism, as muscle is metabolically active tissue. Every pound of muscle in your body burns roughly thirty-five to fifty calories a day to maintain itself. So be patient and go slowly. You'll be rewarded with a faster metabolism and lasting weight loss.

- *Job stress:* Clients' job stress often interfered with their ability to stick to a program. Stress at work kept interfering with efforts to eat the ideal portions and the right types of food. This problem can be magnified for cancer survivors, who often feel under the gun to perform at work. If you are trying to lose weight but just can't stick with an eating or exercise plan, consider whether your job may really be the problem. Do co-workers tempt you with food? Do you often turn to food out of anger, frustration, or sadness? If so, turn to pages 134 to 140 to find ways to reduce job stress.

In addition to overcoming those barriers, when on a program to lose weight you want to develop a system of support. Research completed on breast cancer survivors shows that women who saw a registered dietitian for one-on-one counseling and participated in a group weight-loss program, such as Weight Watchers, lost more weight than women who only participated in individual counseling. So sign up for a group weight-loss class—especially if it's one that includes other cancer survivors—and make sure you receive some one-on-one counseling for nutrition and weight management with someone who works with cancer survivors. This can provide the one-two combination that you need to shed the fat once and for good!

QUIT SMOKING

NEARLY ONE IN every four people smokes despite all the information on its risks, and about half of them will die from the habit. Indeed, more Americans die from tobacco use than from car accidents, suicide, AIDS, homicide, and illegal drug use combined! In addition to cancer, smoking is also associated with heart disease, impotence, infertility, miscarriage, cataracts, hip fractures, and ulcers.

Okay, I had to say it. But the truth is, if you are a survivor of lung, esophageal, larynx, throat, or oral cavity cancer, then you don't need me to preach the evils of tobacco. You know it firsthand. If you needed only fear to help you quit, you would have quit a long time ago!

No, smoking cessation is much tougher than that, as you know. The statistics bear this out. Although 70 percent of smokers want to quit—and although 35 percent attempt to quit each year—fewer than 5 percent actually kick the habit for good. As a survivor, you're all too familiar with odds, and those are not good odds. But, again, as a survivor, you know how to fight and beat the odds—and that's exactly what you need to do! To quit successfully, you first must understand what you're up against. When you try to quit or cut back on smoking, you'll experience physical and psychological withdrawal symptoms that include depression, anger, irritability, insomnia, trouble concentrating, restlessness, headache, fatigue, and increased appetite. These symptoms usually start within a few hours of your last cigarette and peak within seventy-two hours. They may linger for just a few days or for several weeks.

To increase the odds of quitting successfully, choose several quitting methods. Talk to your physician about using nicotine-replacement products, such as the patch or gum, in combination with an antidepressant, which can help alleviate some of the psychological symptoms such as tension and mood changes that can be associated with quitting. Follow up with plenty of support. Ask family and friends to help you quit. If they smoke, ask them not to smoke around you (and not to ask you to take a smoking break with them). Ask them to help alleviate stress during the first week that you quit—as this is the time your withdrawal symptoms will be at their height. Perhaps friends and family can pitch in with household chores. Co-workers might be willing to shoulder some of your workload. (Or, if possible, consider taking a vacation to enable quitting).

Finally, investigate online or phone-based support, such as quit lines. Most states run a free quit line, which will link you with trained counselors who can help design a quitting method for you. Research shows that people who use these quit lines are twice as likely to stop smoking as people who do not. You can find a quit line in your area by calling the American Cancer Society 1-800-ACS-2345.

DEALING WITH CHEMO BRAIN

MANY CANCER SURVIVORS—MYSELF included—experience a range of cognitive limitations when trying to get things done at home and at work. These changes are real. Documented by neuropsychologists, these cognitive problems may be due to direct neurotoxic effects of the chemotherapy agents on our brains that affect the nerve fibers that send messages.

Although experts refer to these limitations as "subtle" deficits, they are far from subtle! They may interfere with your ability to remember names when introduced, phone numbers, addresses, or names of files you just worked on and stored *somewhere* in your computer. You might also experience difficulty multitasking and in focusing your attention for long periods of time.

For me, these cognitive deficits include: not always being able to remember what people tell me, the content of things that I read, or what I plan to do next. I also find that my ability to keep things organized and on track isn't what it used to be. To help overcome these deficits, I met with physician and psychologist specialists and read many studies and texts on neuropsychology. I uncovered a number of helpful strategies that I'd like to share with you. They can help you get a better handle on your memory, organizational skills, and concentration, allowing you to accomplish more without feeling frustrated or fatigued and thus improving your quality of life.

Get enough sleep. Make sure you feel rested after sleeping. The number of hours you sleep are not as important of the quality of your sleep. If you feel refreshed and ready to face the day in the morning, you slept well. If not, you probably did not. Improve your sleep quality by relaxing before bed (some people like to take a warm bath or read a book), making your sleep environment more comfortable by installing better shades on the windows or buying more comfortable pillows, and eliminating noises and other things that wake you up (such as by wearing earplugs to tune out a snoring spouse). If you wake repeatedly at night and can't discern the cause, see a sleep specialist.

Take breaks. When I find myself searching for a file I can't find, I get up from my computer, take a walk, and get a drink of water. These short breaks give my brain a chance to rest and recover. I find that when I return to the task at hand, I feel refreshed, better organized, and more on track.

Work on least interesting or most complex tasks when you are most alert. We all have moments or times of the day when we experience surges and lags in brain power. When you feel "on," tackle the tasks that will require the most out of your brain. When you feel "off," tackle more mindless tasks, such as reading e-mails or your snail mail, writing a simple memo or letter, or making a few phone calls.

Work in a brightly lit room with a window and clock. The lighting can help you stay alert. The clock can help you pace things. Try to allocate a certain amount of time to a given task. Then take a break. The clock in the room can help you keep on track time-wise with that task. If you find you allocated too much time, go on to another task; if you allocated too little time, give yourself another time limit so you can keep going with the task.

Work in a quiet place to minimize distractions. Turn off the ringer on your phone or, if possible, set your phone so calls go directly to voicemail. Put a DO NOT DISTURB sign on your door along with a time interval. Put on a set of headphones to drown out office noise.

Do one thing at a time. When working on the computer, don't answer the phone. When talking on the phone, don't check e-mail.

Keep yourself focused on one thing at a time. Make a list of what needs to get done and in what order. Don't overwhelm yourself, and if you do feel that you are getting hit from all sides, step back and stop all activity for a few minutes and allow yourself to refocus back on the task at hand.

Make the most of your PDA (personal data assistant) or calander. Use it (or a paper calendar or a notebook for the nontechnical among you) to organize tasks. I use a PDA and notebook and still have problems, but they help. Enter tasks according to the deadlines. Give them priority levels: ASAP, Today, Tomorrow, This Week, and When I Can Get to It. Also, write down who, if anyone, is working with you on particular projects.

Schedule tasks in a time frame that will allow you to stay focused. Determine how long you can stay on a task before losing focus, and use that as your time frame before you take a break in your work.

Break up complex tasks into segments. Complete each segment in order, taking breaks after you finish each smaller part of the larger tasks.

Stick to a regular routine. You usually remember to brush your teeth because you do it roughly at the same time of day every day. Try to create many similar routines throughout your day. List all of the tasks that you do every day. Try to do them at the same time of day in the same order. Eventually they will all become a habit and you no longer will need to spend mental energy to *remember* to do them.

Use sticky notes to your advantage. Place small reminders throughout your office to help stay on track. Read these notes out loud, providing visual and auditory input for your memory. Keep a daily to-do list in plain view. Throughout the day, add tasks as they come to mind and check off tasks as you complete them.

Take notes—always. Write down important information. Take notes at meetings or in discussions. Later, if you can't recall a conversation you had with your doctor or with a co-worker, you can check your notes. Although this note taking may at first seem tedious, you'll be happy you did it when you need your notes to jog your memory.

Repeat information and tasks you want to remember. You might sound like a broken record, but this simple trick will help cement that information into your memory. So when your boss asks you to do x, y, and z, just say back to your boss, "You want me to do x, y, and z. I am going to do x, y, and z right now."

Leave yourself a voicemail. Call your phone at work or home, and leave yourself a reminder to do various tasks.

Make lists. Lists are a good way to keep on top of things that need to be done, but allow yourself to not always need to scratch off every item every day. The list is supposed to be helpful to you and not cause you additional stress.

Visualize information you want to remember. Close your eyes and imagine the material, creating a mental picture of the information. For example, if someone is telling you about the next steps on a project, visualize yourself doing each of these steps. Also, use visual tools, such as lists, diagrams, and pictures, to reconstruct the information, translating the spoken word into visual pictures, figures, and charts.

Reduce stress. High levels of stress make it more difficult for you to remember, plan, organize, and stay focused. See pages 138 to 140 for helpful stress-reducing techniques.

Be realistic. You may not be able to keep the same schedule after cancer that you did before cancer. Beg out of unnecessary engagements. Give yourself extra time to complete tasks and modify your work or social requirements to reduce surprises and time and performance pressure. Pace yourself, never taking on more than you can realistically handle.

Slow down. Take time to think about how you want to handle a task or situation. Before your chemo, you probably reacted with the right approach on a regular basis. Now you may need a little time to think about all of your options and choose the most reasonable one before you act.

Acknowledge your mistakes and correct them. You will make mistakes. They happen. Don't try to hide them. Rather, as soon as possible, correct any errors. Acknowledge to others that you may have contributed to confusion or uncertainty. You made a mistake. So what? You're human. Acknowledge it and move on.

If, despite these strategies, your cognitive limitations are an annoyance and/or they impact your quality of life, I recommend you meet with a neuropsychologist, as I have done. He or she can help you work around certain problems by giving you specific suggestions for dealing with the actual deficits uncovered during testing.

Also, talk to your doctor about prescription medication (such as stimulants) that might help. Side effects can include high blood pressure, so talk to your regular doctor before taking these.

REDUCE WORK STRESS

IN THIS SECTION, you will find information and ways you can help with the return to work or volunteer process so you will not have to unnecessarily face leaving a job that you may financially need and want.

The average human being spends half of his or her waking hours at work. It's a big part of our day and contributes greatly to our sense of well-being. On average, roughly 74 percent of cancer survivors younger than age fifty return to work, whereas just 30 percent of those older than age fifty do so.

All of us need to feel productive in some way. It is critical to your self-esteem to maintain a level of productivity similar to that prior to your illness. Returning to work can help reduce stress in other parts of your life. The more satisfaction and success you find at work, the less stressed you feel about other aspects of survivorship. Of course, how you feel about your job depends in part on how you feel in general. Some survivors take off for a month or so during or even for some time after their treatment, until they can mentally and physically get back on their feet. So, although returning to work generally can improve your mental and physical health, don't force yourself to return too soon.

Listen to your body—and your doctor—and return only when you feel ready.

Although many survivors can simply return to work (or may even have never left the job), others have to overcome some obstacles to do so. For example, Elizabeth, age fifty, returned to her job as a nurse right after her diagnosis and treatment for ovarian cancer. She soon realized, however, that she would need a few changes in order to accommodate her reduced energy level. Before her cancer diagnosis, Elizabeth worked the typical twelve-hour shift, one filled with lots of walking to and from patient rooms. After her cancer treatments, this nonstop walking became very tiring for her, so she negotiated with her supervisor to partner with another nurse for half the day. During the other half of the shift, she created patient-education materials, a task she could complete as she sat at a desk. This accommodation allowed Elizabeth to do the job she loved at a pace she could handle.

> ### Survivor Stat
>
> WHILE MORE than 92 percent of cancer survivors do not perceive employment-related problems and are readily assimilated into the workforce, 7.3 percent of cancer survivors say they have experienced job discrimination.

As Elizabeth's story illustrates, you may need to ask your supervisor for some changes for the return to work process to go smoothly. In addition to common physical challenges—such as your work hours, office setup, or whether you work on your feet—you may also have to confront emotional challenges. What are these obstacles? Here are just a few:

- Your boss takes certain resources from you that you always had before you became ill, and tells you that you won't need them now because of your health. For example, your boss might reassign your assistant to another co-worker.
- Your boss and other co-workers voice discriminatory comments such as, "You can't travel anymore now that you have cancer," "We can't have you handle that account because you might not stay on top of it," and "We need you to operate at 100 percent—like you used to."
- Difficulties with health and life insurance matters at work

To reduce that burden, I'd like to share with you some helpful strategies I've developed over the years in helping many different people return to work after battling serious illnesses.

Factors that Impact Return to Work

TWO FACTORS IN particular can affect your return to work. Consider these factors before you return, so you can negotiate for what you may need on day one or before.

What eases your return to work: Positive attitude by co-workers; flexible hours or tasks; a longer time has passed since the end of treatment; support from family, friends, and co-workers.

What complicates your return to work: Manual labor (lifting, standing, walking); long, inflexible work hours; the type of cancer you had, as some types of cancer patients (e.g., testicular cancer) find it easier to return to work than others (e.g., head and neck cancer); the financial need to work.

Use your doctor as your strongest ally. Discuss your plans to return to work with your doctor(s), your family, and your employer. If you have been on leave for an extended period of time, your doctor may need to provide a statement that you are able to return to work, depending on your job and your company's policy. Such a written note should include any work restrictions or limitations you have that protect you from further injury or complication, and any changes that you may need in your environment, such as needing to avoid standing for long periods of time to keep fatigue in check. Your doctor(s) will be able to discuss how to manage symptoms while in the workplace, and may suggest strategies to deal with fatigue, pain, job stress, or other types of challenges you may experience when you return to work. He or she may suggest you start with a reduced schedule, allowing you to slowly develop the strength and stamina needed for full-time work. Follow this advice and use it when discussing your plans with your employer. Use your doctor as the voice of authority that guides your return to work decisions.

Lean on the Americans with Disabilities Act (ADA). This act was signed into law on July 26, 1990. It prohibits private employers, state and local governments, employment agencies, and labor unions from discriminating against qualified individuals with disabilities in job application procedures, hiring, firing, advancement, compensation, job training, and other terms, conditions, and privileges of employment. For the purposes of this law, a person with a disability is described as a person who:

- has a physical or mental impairment that substantially limits one or more major life activities;
- has a record of such an impairment; or
- is regarded as having such impairment.

Given this definition, you may be protected under the ADA. This means you are entitled to a "reasonable accommodation" to help you maintain your job. A reasonable accommodation may include the following: making existing facilities accessible, restructuring your job, modifying your work schedule, reassigning you to a vacant position, or acquiring or modifying equipment or devices to help you work more effectively. These accommodations, however, cannot create an "undue hardship" on the operation of the employer's business. This means that the accommodation must be considered in light of factors such as an employer's size, financial resources, and the nature and structure of its operation. For more information on the Americans with Disabilities Act, go to www.ada.gov or call 1-800-514-0301. This is a government-sponsored Web site and call center that will provide you with the most current information on the ADA.

Lean on the Family and Medical Leave Act (FMLA). This employment law allows people with serious illnesses and their family members to take unpaid leaves of absences from work. Under this act, you are allowed to take up to twelve weeks of unpaid leave within one year. You may renew this leave once a year, every year. Although your paychecks will stop, your employee benefits (e.g. your life and/or health insurance) continue during your time. You need not take your twelve-week leave all at once. You are allowed to take your time in blocks of time, such as several hours a day. (You may need to take an alternative temporary position if variable hours cannot be accommodated in your current position.) For more information on this law and how it applies to you, go to the U.S. Government, Department of Labor, Employment Standards Administration's Web site, www .dol.gov/esa/whd/fmla, or call 1-866-4-USA-DOL.

Take frequent breaks. Take a walk or sit outside during a lunch break, if you can. If you feel yourself becoming anxious or overwhelmed, take a break. Also, think about the expectations you have for yourself. What standards are you trying to live up to? Are they realistic? Share your feelings with friends and family outside of work. Finally, find ways to reward yourself for doing all you do. It may sound silly, but nurture yourself and be proud of your efforts.

Manage fatigue. This is an area where your doctor can help. You may need to schedule routine breaks to rest before you become very tired, schedule the most important tasks for earlier in the day when you are fresher, or work reduced hours until you can gradually increase the time as you are able to gain strength; you may also need to do something to help you get a better night of rest. Become aware of your body and listen to it.

Manage pain. The same holds true for pain management as it does for fatigue management. Listen to your body and pace yourself. Talk to your doctor and work out a reasonable plan that makes the most sense for you. It may be helpful to make certain accommodations to minimize effects of your environment (e.g., a headset may be worn instead of using a handheld phone, to reduce the stress on your arm or shoulder). Many physical and occupational therapists can help with this.

Also, consider taking a nonsteroidal anti-inflammatory agent (NSAID), as research shows these pain-killing medications are just as effective as strong opioids but are not sedating. Depending on the type of your cancer and other factors, a pain specialist can review with you a number of medical approaches that can help control pain, such as nerve blocks that destroy the nerve pathway signaling the pain (called *neurolytic blocks*).

Communicate your needs. With good communication skills (such as the ones you learned in chapter 3) you can get many of the accommodations at work that you need simply by laying them out and relate them to how they can help you complete your essential work tasks. They do need to be reasonable. Do this with your supervisor and the person who would be responsible at work for actually implementing these accommodations, if they are not the same person. Many times, for example, your office manager may work in conjunction with your supervisor to modify your work schedule to allow you a rest period as well as time off for doctor's appointments or other treatments, create a workspace with less distractions, or permit the shifting of some of your responsibilities to support staff. Approach the negotiation with an open mind and try to be as realistic as possible, given your employer, and your perspectives. Use these pointers when communicating these needs with such colleagues:

- Make an appointment to speak with your supervisor; do not rely on chance meetings to help you plan.
- Allow your supervisor time to check out company policies and procedures.
- Treat him or her as another collaborator in your achievement of quality health care and enhanced quality of life.
- Without disclosing more than necessary or comfortable, provide some insight on what you are experiencing at work and what your condition means for you.
- Keep careful and thorough notes of the meetings to not only serve as reminders of what was agreed to, but also as a way to help you focus on your needs for success at work.
- Be prepared to educate your employer. Think about how little you knew about what your condition meant before it happened to you.
- Bring a written doctor's note to the meeting. It puts a third party with authority between you and your supervisor to objectively point out limitations and accommodation options that may help.
- If you are having difficulty coming to an agreement, ask to meet with your supervisor and a representative from human resources. Remember how emotions impacted your ability to hear and understand information provided to you from your doctor or other health-care providers. You may be experiencing some of those responses now. Also, your supervisor may have some feelings about your condition that is affecting how he or she is responding to you.
- Tell your co-workers about your work expectations and any modifications you and your supervisor have made to your schedule. You may have shared more details of your condition or illness with your supervisor than you wish to share with your colleagues. Without those additional pieces of information, it may be difficult for your colleagues to understand the modifications you need. Again, let your supervisor lead that discussion and do not discuss the rationale with your colleagues unless you feel comfortable doing so.

Talk about your plans with your family. Our fast-paced society already makes balancing work and family a challenge, but when you toss cancer into the mix, things become even more complicated. It helps if you share your goals and expectations with your family and you plot out with them a schedule for yourself. Then, once you get into a routine, go back and discuss that schedule with them to see how it may need to change. Again, communication and patience are key. Plan adequate rest for yourself, and build in relaxing time with your family as well.

Get help. If you can afford it, hire outside help to manage some of the household chores for your initial return to work. This need not be an expensive endeavor or a permanent situation. Consider paying high school kids to cut your grass or do other household tasks. Advertise in your local paper or church bulletin for a handyman or household helper to get at some of the tasks that need to be done, but that are taxing upon your time and energy.

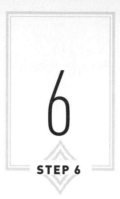

STEP 6

See Life Through More Optimistic Eyes

WHEN PAUL LEARNED he had lymphocytic leukemia, he only wanted one thing: to survive. His search for the best tests, doctors, and treatments kept him so busy that the seriousness of the illness didn't really sink in. It was some months after his initial diagnosis—after treatment began to kick in according to his blood tests—that a complex bundle of emotions set in. He became sad and reflective. He realized his life would never again be the same. He noticed feeling more tired. It seemed as if he couldn't remember things as well as he did before his treatments. Sometimes, he couldn't concentrate for long periods of time. Work was a major source of stress for him, but he could not just quit: he needed the job for lots of reasons.

Yes, he felt fortunate that things were moving along on the right track, but he also felt out of touch with his life, his routine, his family and friends, and even his joy of playing golf. His inability to remember names and things he was just told frustrated him. He worried before each medical visit. Sadness, anger, frustration, and anxiety seemed like constant companions.

To help Paul move on, I taught him many of the same psychological techniques that I had taught police officers, firefighters, and others who had survived life-threatening situations, such as shootouts, or observed the worst of humanity, such as wife beatings or child abuse or even childhood killings. These simple techniques have also helped me manage my stress and get back on track. They helped Paul, and they will help you, too. First,

Hope vs. Realism

YOU'VE PROBABLY HEARD that hope can keep you going. It's true, but only to a point. If you simply hope that, over time, you'll feel better, your emotional outlook won't change all that much. As survivors, we can all benefit from a certain degree of realistic optimism. It helps us realize that, yes, things can get better over time, but only if we take steps to make them better. Just hoping that things will change very rarely results in change. We must work on the best ways to achieve these goals to get on with what we need to and improve our lives. That's what I mean by realistic optimism. Yes, be upbeat and look forward to better days, but also realize the journey is not easy. We need to make things happen.

however, you must realize that whatever you are feeling—no matter how negative (or positive)—is completely normal.

If you feel angry or frustrated that your co-workers and boss expect more out of you now that your initial treatments have ended, even though you are doing the best you can, you're normal. If you feel stressed about medical bills that keep coming in each time you go for a consultation for something concerning your health, you're normal. If you had to reduce many of the extra things at work or in your leisure time, you're normal. If you worry that any day the cancer might come back, you're normal. If you feel indecisive about taking on new responsibilities, planning social events, or scheduling appointments because you don't know whether you'll have the energy to follow through, you're normal. If you feel guilty that you survived when you hear about others who haven't, you are normal. (And, conversely, if you are simply happy to be alive, well, that's normal, too!)

All of these emotions are part of what we call the "stress response," our reaction to threatening situations. Every human on the planet experiences stress. From demanding work schedules and long commutes to noisy dogs and clanging construction, stress is a constant in life. Yet, stress may feel *more intense* to cancer survivors. The same pro-inflammatory cytokines and other immunity markers that helped our bodies to fight the cancer are also involved in such negative emotions and symptoms as pain, fatigue, anxiety, and depression.

When you're exposed to stress, the adrenal glands release the stress hormones epinephrine and norepinephrine. These chemicals increase our heart rate, blood pressure, and breathing rate; dilate pupils; slow digestion; and shuttle blood away from the digestive tract and to the working muscles, preparing you to fight or run. The hypothalamus, a part of our brain, also triggers the release of corticosteroids. In the short term, these chemicals combat inflammation, promote healing, and initiate fat storage to ready your body to fight off the threat. But when this stress response doesn't go away—as it sometimes does not with cancer—it can contribute to poor health.

> ## Survivor Stat
>
> AN ONLINE survey recently conducted by the Lance Armstrong Foundation (LAF) of 1,020 cancer survivors (ages 18 to 75) reveals that nearly half struggle with non-medical needs, such as emotional distress. In fact, they report that they experience more distress over these emotional issues than the physical ramifications of cancer. A startling 70 percent of survivors report feeling depressed, a full two years after their final treatments.

You can take many steps to de-stress your environment by talking with your spouse, your kids, and your boss to try to straighten out problems so they do not resurface. You can also deal with stress from the inside—how you react to it.

Stress can affect cancer. Prolonged stress elevates such chemicals as cortisol, which, in turn, reduces the number of white blood cells and cytokines, and hinders the functioning of lymphocytes. These biological changes reduce the body's ability to fight cancer growth. It's not that stress causes the cancer, but it might make it worse (and it certainly can make you feel worse).

When stress persists, you not only feel negative emotions, such as fear and sadness, but you may also experience physical symptoms, such as headaches and other aches and pains in muscles. The way you experience stress can disrupt your sleep, make pain worse, and contribute to fatigue—some of the very concerns that may stress you out in the first place! Also the negative emotions that stem from stress can cloud your judgment, preventing you from making the best decisions about your care, family, or work.

> ## Survivor Stat
>
> PEOPLE WHO respond to stress with a higher degree of anger are 1.5 times more likely to have a heart attack than people who respond to stress with a low level of anger.

Here's the good news. Just as stress can cause these negative changes, stress-reduction techniques can reverse things. In a study of women who survived early-stage breast cancer, stress-reduction techniques, along with positive thinking, improved lymphocyte activity, thereby improving the women's likelihood of fighting off new cancer cell growth. The simple techniques you'll find in this chapter will help you to reduce stress, improve your mood, and learn to see cancer survival more positively—as a chance to live your life anew.

THE STRESS OF SURVIVAL

I'VE COUNSELED MANY survivors in my private practice, in support groups, and over the Internet. Most tell me that they expected to feel strong emotions during their battle with cancer. They didn't, however, expect the anger, depression, frustration, guilt, and fear to linger so long after treatment. There are also many survivors who do not experience these feelings. That does not mean there is something wrong with you. Coping with cancer is an individual thing. Everyone handles it differently.

The mind-set after cancer is similar to the mind-set after any near-death experience. Before my brain tumor, I served as a behavioral health consultant for the Washington, D.C. police and firefighters as well as for the U.S. Secret Service. In this role, I often counseled men and women who had survived life-threatening situations.

> ## Survivor Stat
>
> IN STUDIES completed on patients with rectal, breast, testicular, esophageal, or prostate cancer, survivors reported better quality of life than did members of the general population. "The experience of cancer" may induce a conscious awareness that leads to a positive appreciation of everyday life.

They had been shot at or hit by cars. They had wrestled suspects to the ground and pulled their weapons. They had survived high-speed chases and witnessing the death of their partners to gunfire.

After such events, many could not sleep or eat for days. Memories of the incident made them feel hyper, tense, and sad. They became irritable with loved ones and fellow workers. They would avoid certain places where the events took place. The sounds of a slamming car door or other sudden loud noises would trigger startle reactions. Some also felt that they could have prevented what happened if they only did something differently, such as helped their partner earlier or called for assistance or tried to disarm a suspect. When this persisted for more than a month, it was clear to me that they were suffering from a condition known as post-traumatic stress disorder (PTSD).

Many cancer survivors experience features of the same condition. As with the officers and others that I have counseled, cancer survivors often relive different aspects of the diagnosis, treatment, and other aspects of the cancer experience over and over. Just as police officers worry about another shooting, cancer survivors worry about the threat of a recurrence. We hear about a survivor whose cancer returned or, even worse, who died. Initially, the news gives us goose bumps. Then come the thoughts: "When will it be my turn?" "That could be me." "Did he have the same type of cancer I had?" "How long will my good health last?" We feel edgy and tense, flinching at the slightest loud noise, tossing and turning at night, dreaming about new tumor growth, hospitalization, and surgeries. Each time we anticipate negative consequences, such as a doctor's visit or a follow-up MRI or mammogram, these negative thoughts trigger a stress response. This is called "anticipatory stress" or "anticipatory anxiety," and it elevates stress hormones.

The day you learned you had cancer was the initial stressor that can set off the post traumatic stress disorder. You may not have realized you were under stress at first. You simply went on autopilot and did what you needed to do to survive. Now, although many of the big decisions and treatments are over with, the stress remains. It is important to emphasize that not every cancer survivor experiences this. Also, the longer you are a survivor the more likely these things pass.

SIMPLE WAYS TO FEEL BETTER

LET'S GO BACK to Paul. To reduce stress and feel better emotionally, he first reduced his workload and stopped working eighteen-hour days. He took control of his schedule and reduced the number of meetings to a small, manageable number. He began communicating with people more by e-mail and reduced the number of phone calls and phone messages, asking people to e-mail him instead.

He also worked on changing his reaction to stress. Paul realized he could not eliminate all stress in his world. For some of it, he would have to learn how to deal with it differently. Fortunately, the techniques I showed him really helped.

In addition to using the relaxation techniques you'll soon learn, Paul

Do You Have Post-Traumatic Stress Disorder?

IF THE FOLLOWING symptoms persist for longer than one month, you may have PTSD. See a clinical psychologist, social worker, or psychiatrist trained in using cognitive behavior therapy techniques, perhaps along with medications that have been scientifically shown to help this problem. Your health professional will enable you to talk about the situation, reduce your mental (fear, guilt), physical (heart rate, muscle tension, sleep disturbance), and behavioral (avoidance) reactions to the stress, better understand the situation, and move on. The symptoms include:

- Unwanted thoughts about surgery, radiation, or drug treatment you have undergone
- Insomnia
- Irritability
- Poor concentration
- Increased startle reactions
- Avoidance of reminders of the cancer (such as avoiding going to hospitals because they trigger thoughts of the cancer)

now tunes out stress by listening to music, reading, talking to family and friends, sitting on his deck, and taking walks. Over time, you'll find your own relaxation methods, just as Paul did. When you combine them with the techniques from this chapter, you'll get even better results.

Stress-Reducing Tactic #1: Keep a Stress Diary

To reduce stress, you first must notice when you are under stress and pinpoint what's causing it. Only then can you either eliminate the stressor or try to change your reaction to it. Sometimes stress is obvious; other times, it's more subtle. Pay attention to the following mental, physical, and behavioral signs of stress.

Mental signs of stress: negative thoughts and emotions, including anger, anxiety, and sadness

Physical signs of stress: Muscle tension, stomach upset, chest tightness, headache, fatigue, racing heartbeat

Behavioral signs of stress: Snapping at your kids, pounding your fists on a table, muttering obscenities under your breath, driving aggressively, desperately needing a "fix" of an unhealthy food not in your diet plan

We all deal with stress in our own, unique way. Your thoughts, physical signs, and behavior may differ from what I've included in the symptoms list, so pay careful attention to your thoughts, sensations, and actions to determine your personal stress style.

Once you get in touch with these signs of stress, you can determine what triggers your stress. To do so, keep a stress diary for a few weeks (consult the sample stress diary on page 148, for its suggested format). When you notice physical, mental, and behavioral signs of stress, write down the date, time, triggering event, what thoughts that ran through your mind, and how you handled the stress. If you don't know exactly what triggered your stress response, jot down the circumstances that had occurred during the half hour before you noticed you were under stress.

For example, when you notice yourself tensing up, you might write down a conversation you had with your boss just moments earlier. Or, perhaps you tensed up because you couldn't remember what you needed to do next at work. Keep in mind that some sources of stress are external (people, deadlines, traffic) whereas others stem from internal sensations (such as pain, fatigue) or belief systems and thought patterns (such as fear, disappointment, and frustration).

Keep notes in your stress diary for a few weeks. Then take a look at your diary. Look for common stress triggers. These are the situations that you'll want to deal with first. For example, if one person repeatedly said something to you that triggered numerous stress responses during the three weeks you kept the diary, you'll want to confront that person!

Also look carefully at how you interpreted the situation. As I mentioned earlier, we can't always change the situation. Sometimes, we must change how we *respond to* the situation. You'll soon learn some effective techniques for doing so. For now, however, use your stress diary to get a handle on the internal thoughts and feelings that may be triggering stress. In your diary, look at the thoughts that ran through your mind. What did you say to yourself? Was it a reflexive reaction that made you feel worse? Circle

Stress Diary

DATE:	STRESSFUL EVENT:
Where and when did the event occur?	
What made the event stressful?	
What were your reactions?	
Body (e.g., heart pounding, muscles tense, hands sweating)	
Thoughts (e.g., He/she should not treat me this way, I should not have to deal with this.)	
What feelings did you experience (e.g., anger, frustration, fear, fatigue:	
Rate the intensity of the feeling on a 1 to 10 scale.	

(no stress)	1	2	3	4	5	6	7	8	9	10	(worst stress)

How did you handle the event?	
What would you do differently if it happens again?	
What was your reaction to the stressor (your behavior and thoughts)?	

any thoughts that you think may have caused your stress response. Doing so will help you later, when you get to stress-reduction tactic #4.

Stress-reducing tactic #2: Stop the stressor

Your diary will give you a better idea of what causes your stress, allowing you to reduce some of the stressors in your life. For example, when Linda, a brain tumor survivor, first returned to work after her cancer treatments, she found her previous job responsibilities overwhelming. Also, her co-workers seemed a little distant, making her feel uncomfortable.

To address the situation, she sat down with her supervisor and listed the major tasks of her job. Together, she and her supervisor talked about each task, with Linda indicating whether or not she could still perform it. They also talked about some reasonable accommodations her supervisor could make—such as allowing Linda to occasionally work from home to help make completion of the necessary tasks of the job possible. After hashing out the essential job responsibilities, Linda settled back into work. She also spoke to her co-workers, explaining that she felt stronger every day but that she could not perform some job functions in the time frame she had before her surgery. After addressing these issues, she felt much more comfortable at work.

You won't always be able to eliminate the stressors in your life, but it is always worth a try. Below you will find some common stressors of cancer survivorship along with possible ways to reduce them:

Stressor: A family member tells you she is tired of your talking about how you feel.
Solution: Discuss your feelings with her. Say, "I know you are tired of all this, but I do need to talk to someone. Can you help me work something out here?" Also, "Let's work some compromise; it must be frustrating for you to hear this all the time."

Stressor: You feel depressed.
Solution: Try taking a walk, exercising, or doing something enjoyable that you have not done for a while. Quite often, simply doing something we enjoy really does work. Even if you have to force yourself to get up out of the chair and go to a movie or out to dinner or onto the golf course (or wherever you usually feel happy), just do it!

Stressor: You are expressing concern over a deadline at work and someone tells you to "just suck it up."
Solution: Talk with your co-worker and ask him in a very firm tone to not talk you that way and that it makes you more stressed when he makes those types of comments.

Stressor: You forget what you are about to do at work or home.
Solution: Make a list of the things you plan to do, as soon as you think about them, and carry this list with you everywhere.

Stressor: You have been invited out to a social gathering, but feel awkward because you have not been out much since your cancer treatment ended; you wonder what people might say to you.
Solution: Make a list of the questions that you think others might ask you. Think of how you might answer them. Rehearse the responses. Also, you do not need to always answer people's questions directly. If you are uncomfortable, have a general response ready, such as "I'm doing much better, thank you for your concern," then turn the conversation to a more comfortable topic.

Stressor: Yet another medical bill comes in the mail. This time, the lab is questioning whether your insurance will cover the claim and they are asking you to pay the full amount.
Solution: If you are upset with the bill, set it down and take a walk, or talk to a friend before you try to deal with it. Keeping yourself calm is the best way to deal with bill collectors. First of all, don't assume they are correct. Make a call to gather some facts. Perhaps the claim was lost or not even submitted to the insurance company. Second, if you are not able to make the call yourself, ask a family member or friend for help. Your insurance company will only release information if you're on the line, so ask the friend or family member to listen in on another phone and to chime in at your signal. If, in the end, the bill is your responsibility, work out a payment plan that is manageable for you.

If you experience a stressor not on the previous list, use the problem-solving strategy from chapter 2 to generate possible solutions. Keep in mind that you cannot eliminate or reduce every stressor. In that case, you must learn how to cope with the stress by changing your reaction to it (see tactic #4).

Stress-Reducing Tactic #3: Refocus Your Thoughts

You might think that certain people and events cause your stress. They can *contribute to* it, but they don't *cause* it. Your thoughts and beliefs about the situations around you make you feel what you do. Almost every minute of our lives, a constant barrage of chatter takes place in our minds. Some of us talk to ourselves out loud. All of us talk to ourselves silently—all the time. This self-talk plays a significant role in how you describe and interpret the world. Thoughts and beliefs work like a filter that colors the world you see. You can change the impact of the stressor by monitoring and changing the filter (your thoughts) that exists between your encounter with the stressor and your reaction to it. The goal is to adjust your outlook to one that enables you to deal effectively with the stressor.

If your thoughts are unrealistic, then you experience the symptoms of stress. Unrealistic, stress-producing thoughts are often based on one of the following:

- outright *misperceptions* ("When the airplane's wing shakes, I know it is going to fall off.")
- perfectionistic *shoulds, oughts,* and *musts* ("I ought to keep quiet rather than upset anyone.")

For example, the stress-producing thought "I can't do anything right" does not accurately portray reality. No person on this earth does everything wrong. You might have bad days during which you make more mistakes than usual, but you don't make mistakes all the time. Here's yet another stress-producing thought: "I must always be able to get all my work done under the deadline—everyone else does." The words *should* and *must* allow little possibility of flaw, failure or events that you can not control. When the inevitable occurs (you have an off day or you are given an unrealistic deadline), by indulging in such thoughts you indict yourself as being entirely ineffective, all on the basis of a single incident.

At the root of most irrational thinking is the assumption that things are done *to* you: "*That* really got me down. . . . *She* makes me nervous. . . . *Places* like that scare me. . . . *Being lied to* makes me see red." In reality, however,

nothing is done *to* you

Your own thoughts, *directed and controlled by you,* create stress, anger,

Thought Refocusing Examples

USE THE FOLLOWING examples to generate ideas on how to refocus your thoughts.

Situation: Someone you know died of cancer.
Initial thought: "I'm going to be next."
Refocused thought: "I'm taking good care of myself. I am thriving. I am here for a reason, to help others."

Situation: A collection agency calls regarding the $30,000 you owe a hospital for your cancer treatments.
Initial thought: "Oh, not again. How am I going to pay this?"
Refocused thought: "I will call them right now, schedule a meeting with the head of hospital billing, and discuss my financial situation. Maybe we can work out a payment plan."

Situation: You feel so tired you can't make it through the afternoon without a nap.
Initial thought: "The cancer must be back."
Refocused thought: "I had a hard day. I need to slow down. I'll take a walk, have a drink of water, and will feel much better."

Situation: Your partner initiates sexual foreplay but you would rather wash the dishes.
Initial thought: "My partner is going to leave me."
Refocused thought: "I'll explain to him how the cancer treatments have affected my sex drive. Maybe I can please him in other ways."

Situation: Your partner wants to go out to a movie, but you want to stay home.
Initial thought: "I am no fun anymore."
Refocused thought: "We went out a few days ago and we both had a great time. I am just too tired tonight. I need to let her know."

When you swap positive thoughts for negative thoughts, you must choose a thought that you really believe. You also might need to follow up with a behavior, such as explaining your situation with the person, as in the last example. This approach often seems contrived at first, especially when using your diary to reconstruct events that have already taken place. You need only practice with your diary a few times, however, before you are ready to try the technique in real time.

As you catch yourself reflexively saying these stress-producing thoughts to yourself, force yourself to come up with alternative stress-reducing thoughts. The more often you do this, the easier and more natural it becomes. You will begin to think and feel more positive. Keep in mind that the goal isn't to feel positive and happy all the time. There will be times when you have every right in the world to feel angry, sad, or frustrated. This process, however, will help to separate stressors you can do something about from stressors you can't do anything about, easing those negative emotions and helping you to see the world in a more positive light.

and tension. Say, an event happens. You experience this event A, engage in self-talk B, and then experience an emotion C resulting from the self-talk. A does not cause C; B causes C. Emotions have little to do with actual events. If your self-talk is unrealistic, you create the unpleasant emotions for yourself; they have not been imposed upon you by the event. A psychologist named Albert Ellis coined this chain of events the "A-B-Cs" of our responses to the world around us. Understanding its dynamics is a helpful way of keeping our feelings in check . . . giving us perspective.

The good news is that you can change stress-producing self-talk. Doing so can decrease your negative emotions and relieve the stress and symptoms that often accompany these emotions. To modify stress-producing thoughts, follow these steps:

1. Look over your stress diary, noticing the facts of an event when you felt stressed.
2. Look at the thoughts that ran through your mind during and just after the event. Pay particular attention to your subjective value judgments, assumptions, beliefs, predictions, and worries.

3. Dispute the irrational self-talk identified in step 2. To do this, ask yourself:
   - Is there any real support for this thought?
   - What is the worst thing that could happen to me?
4. Substitute more positive self-talk.

Stress-Reducing Tactic #4: Relaxation

There are many ways to relax, including meditation, yoga, and exercise. One of the simplest methods to learn, however, is something called *progressive muscular relaxation*. It's so simple you can teach it to yourself; no therapist needed!

Progressive muscular relaxation does exactly as it sounds. Starting at your feet and progressing up your body to your head, you systematically tense and then relax specific muscle groups. As your muscles relax, so will your mind, reducing stress. Progressive muscle relaxation counteracts your physiological stress response and can help you become more aware of how your body experiences tension and stress. This technique allows you to reduce the tension before it becomes excessive.

It can help you to:

- Decrease muscle tension
- Enhance productivity
- Improve decision-making
- Reduce fatigue
- Increase alertness
- Improve sleep
- Lower stress hormone levels
- Lower blood pressure

As you perform the exercise, focus on the sensations you experience when your body shifts from tension to relaxation. Eventually, as you become more adept at the technique, you will be able to relax your muscles without tensing them. As this becomes easier and easier, you'll be able to notice muscle tension and then simply tell your body to relax—and it will listen! Let's begin.

Sit in a comfortable chair. Breathe deeply for a few minutes. Close your eyes, but do not fall asleep. Tense your feet and calves by flexing your feet, tightening your calves, and firming your upper legs. Hold for a count of five. As you hold, notice what this muscle tension feels like. After a count of five, exhale as you release the tension. Your leg muscles will now feel more relaxed. Notice this sensation. Now, move up your legs to your knees and thighs. Straighten your knees and squeeze your thighs together. Hold for a count of five, and then exhale and release. Now your legs should feel even more relaxed.

You will continue in this way, systematically moving up your body.

As you practice progressive muscle relaxation, always hold the tension in your muscles for five seconds before releasing, but do not tense your muscles to the point of pain. Focus on how your muscles feel both when tense and when relaxed. Throughout the exercise, take slow, deep, regular abdominal breaths.

Use the following guide to aid you in your relaxation practice.

1. Feet and Calves
   - Flex the feet by pulling your toes toward your knees.
   - Contract your calf muscles.
   - Tighten your upper legs.
   - Hold five seconds.
   - Relax the muscles.

2. Knees and Upper Thighs
   - Straighten your knees and squeeze your legs together toward the midline of your body.
   - Contract your thigh muscles.
   - Hold five seconds.
   - Relax the muscles.

3. Buttocks and Abdomen
   - Tighten your buttocks, squeezing them inward and upward.
   - Press your naval in toward your spine and contract all of your abdominal muscles.
   - Hold five seconds.
   - Relax the muscles.

4. Upper Back
   - Draw your shoulder blades toward the midline of your body.
   - Contract the muscles across your upper back.

- Hold five seconds.
- Relax the muscles.

5. Arms
   - Turn your palms face down.
   - Flex your fingers back.
   - Raise and straighten your arms.
   - Hold five seconds.
   - Relax the muscles.

6. Chin, Neck, and Shoulders
   - Press your chin against your chest.
   - Draw your shoulders up toward your ears.
   - Hold five seconds.
   - Relax the muscles.

7. Teeth and Facial Muscles
   - Clench your jaws.
   - Turn the corners of your mouth up into a tight smile.
   - Wrinkle your nose and tightly squeeze shut your eyes.
   - Raise your eyebrows and crease your browline.
   - Wrinkle your forehead.
   - Hold five seconds.
   - Relax the muscles.

Once you've reached your head, allow a feeling of relaxation to flow throughout your body, starting at your head, drifting over your face, moving down the back of your neck and shoulders, through your arms, chest, and abdomen, and down through your buttocks, thighs, knees, and feet. Continue breathing deeply and slowly. Notice how your muscles feel in this relaxed state. Try to memorize this sensation. Eventually, with practice, you'll be able to return to this relaxed state more and more quickly.

Once you relax, you won't want to move! Be gentle with your body. Return to normal activity with slow, gradual movements. Wiggle your fingers and toes. Rotate your head. Roll your shoulders and stretch. Then open and focus your eyes.

For best results, practice progressive muscle relaxation at least three times per week for fifteen minutes each session. These practice sessions will help reduce your overall level of muscle tension and relax rapidly. As

The Importance of Deep Breathing

BEFORE READING THE next paragraph, close your eyes and bring your awareness inside. Notice what parts of your torso expand and contract as you breathe. Then open your eyes.

If you are like most people, only your chest rises and falls with each inhalation and exhalation. This type of shallow breathing only brings oxygen to the upper lungs, leaving the middle and lower lungs unfilled. Not only can shallow breathing increase fatigue (after all, you're not inhaling as much oxygen as you could), it also can trigger anxiety. Shallow chest breathing mimics the same rapid breathing of the fight or flight response, creating a chronic stress response in the body. When you breathe shallowly, you actually must tense up a number of muscles as you inhale and exhale.

To relax, you must breathe deeply and slowly. Babies breathe this way naturally. Their bellies rise and fall with each breath. As we age, however, we forget how to breathe! During your progressive muscle relaxation sessions, try to breathe with your belly. In the beginning, you might place a hand on your tummy to encourage yourself to inhale deeply. Eventually, with practice, belly breathing will become second nature—and you'll feel relaxed all day long as a result.

you gain mastery over the technique, you will be able to feel relaxed just by thinking about feeling relaxed. Before each practice session, write down the date and time and rate your current level of tension on a scale from 0 (no tension) to 10 (the worst tension you have ever experienced). Following the exercise, re-rate your tension level. This will help you keep track of your results, fueling your motivation to stick with it.

Stress-Reduction Tactic #5: Write a Letter to Yourself

Journal keeping has positive effects on health and emotions. Many survivors report that expressing their feelings, even by writing them to themselves, elevates their mood, improves physical symptoms such as fatigue and pain, and reduces the need for further treatment.

To do it, write continuously about your deepest thoughts and feelings for about twenty minutes per day. Don't worry about grammar or spelling. Don't edit yourself or try to make it sound good. Just write. You can use an old-fashioned pen and paper, or type up your notes at a computer. Use whatever method allows you to capture your thoughts, feelings, and emotions with the least effort.

To get started, consider writing about the following:

- Your feelings about a recurrence
- Your frustrations at work or home
- Your new limitations; what you can no longer do
- Your new goals in life
- What the experience of cancer means to you
- What cancer has taught you
- Any good cancer has brought to your life
- What you wish your spouse, friends, and kids understood about you, but you are too afraid to tell them
- What you have not done with your life that you would like to

Stress-Reduction Tactic #6: Consider Medication

Radiation and chemotherapy can literally change the human brain, reducing levels of the feel-good brain chemical serotonin. When levels of this chemical run too low, you feel depressed, experience insomnia, and tend to overeat. Many of the prescription medications used to treat depression boost levels of this brain chemical. This can happen with any cancer.

Some survivors do not want to take any additional medications, even if these medications will help. I understand. I've been there. After poisoning your body with chemotherapy, you probably simply want to cleanse yourself of any and all drugs. That's understandable.

That said, taking an antidepressant, even for a short while, can help boost your mood and get you out of bed or that funk, and out experiencing life again. It might

> ## *Survivor Stat*
>
> ACCORDING TO several studies, cancer survivors who express their feelings and emotions visit doctors and hospitals less often, are healthier overall, and experience fewer feelings of sadness and isolation than survivors who don't express their feelings. If you don't feel comfortable talking about your feelings with someone face-to-face, explore Internet discussion groups.

give you the boost you need to put the other techniques suggested in this chapter to work for you.

For example, Susan, a thirty-five-year-old cancer survivor I know, really did not want to take medication to deal with the mood changes and fatigue she experienced after her radiation treatments. Although she recognized that the medication might help, she told me that she had taken enough medications already. The steroids she took during her radiation treatments had kept her up all night, made her moody, and caused her to gain lots of weight because she could not stop eating. So, in lieu of antidepressants, Susan started exercising, meditating, and refocusing her thoughts. After a few months of this, however, she had lingering feelings of stress and periodic despair. At that point, she decided she had tried her best and continued exercising but also filled a prescription for an antidepressant.

I bumped into Susan about three months after she began taking the antidepressant. She told me that she felt great! She also mentioned she had much more energy than before.

If you decide to pursue antianxiety or antidepressant medication, keep the following in mind:

- You may need to try a few before you find one that works for you.
- If you experience side effects (such as lowered sexual desire or weight gain), a lower dosage or different medication may solve the problem.
- If you notice side effects or your mood does not improve, call your doctor.
- If you start taking a medication, consult your doctor before stopping.
- You may find that the benefits of the medication are only apparent when you have a consistent level of the drug in your body. This means that you may need to take it indefinitely.

Consult the table on in Appendix B to learn the common side effects of medications used to treat anxiety and depression.

A BETTER FUTURE

FOLLOWING MY CANCER treatment, I knew I needed to move on, but I still felt pretty down. I lived in fear. I didn't know whether the treatments really worked or for how long, I had read that, even if an MRI does not reveal cancer, millions of hidden cancer cells may still be dividing in your brain. I wondered how much time I really had left. I worried whether I would be able to support my family financially, continue to work, and to fulfill other responsibilities. One day, I was talking to my son Andy about all of this. He looked at me and firmly said, "Dad, isn't it time you stop this pity fest?"

His comment startled me and helped me to see the negative filter my internal thoughts were placing on the world around me. I realized it was time to move on.

Now, when I start to worry, I change my internal self-talk to something more positive. It has really helped me to begin to live my life after cancer. Thoughts still come and go, and some days are better than others, but these approaches do help.

I realized that I needed to redefine many aspects of my life. I was not the same person. I decided to get to know and accept the new me and move on. I now relax more than I used to and talk even more directly to people, I try to get the point, letting them know my views and listening to theirs, but moving the discussion to the bottom line much faster.

I also now realize that I am fortunate. Now, after the cancer, I find I can more easily put life in perspective. After the cancer, I reevaluated my workload, opting to spend more time at home. I take more time for what matters to me most: my wife and my children and grandchild. I also allocate time to better understand cancer survivorship from a scientific point of view, so I can help others in my situation translate this work into useful answers to the question, "now what?"

I feel blessed that I've been around for major family milestones, such as the wedding of my daughter, the graduation of my son from college, my grandson's birth, and so on. I am looking forward to the graduation from high school of my youngest daughter. I'm optimistic about the future and excited to leave my unique mark on the world. I know, you too, will soon find yourself in the same place.

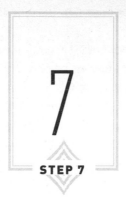

7

STEP 7

Create Your Future

THROUGHOUT THIS BOOK, we've focused on the challenges that many of us face after cancer. Think of the challenges to your survivorship journey as a series of hurdles on a track. Getting the quality heath care you need for a problem that crops up may represent one hurdle for you. Workplace accommodations, another. Lingering fatigue and a focus on preventing other noncancer illnesses, still others. Throughout this book, you've learned a series of strategies to help you overcome those hurdles. These strategies provide the tools you need—the track shoes, muscle power, technique, and spring in your step—to leap over and clear these hurdles.

Cancer survivorship is a journey, one that takes you down the track of life, springing over one hurdle at a time. With each hurdle that you clear, your life will become more and more healthy, meaningful, and positive.

So far, you've learned how to get the health-care system to work for you, choose the best providers and communicate with them more effectively, make better decisions, reduce stress, improve your lifestyle and quality of life, maximize support, and much, much more. Although you now have the tools you need to clear these hurdles to better health and quality of life, you still need to develop a plan to put those tools into action. Your plan will help you implement the right training strategies so you can jump higher, sailing over a particular hurdle. Each hurdle may require a slightly different training regimen. Do the right training and this journey won't feel as challenging!

You may feel tempted to focus on several hurdles at once. Try to resist this urge. Imagine that track again for a minute. Think about what would happen if you stacked all of those hurdles one on top of another. They would turn into a tall, insurmountable wall, one that no human on the planet could surmount. On the other hand, if you evenly space those hurdles a good distance apart and focus only on clearing one hurdle at a time, they suddenly don't look so insurmountable! So I encourage you to think of your survivorship journey in this way. You have what it takes to clear each hurdle if you focus on jumping over just one hurdle at a time.

You can't possibly change every aspect of your life at once. More important, you probably don't need to. As you read along chapter by chapter, you may have thought to yourself from time to time, "I'm doing just fine in that area." Other times, you may have thought, "Wow, I really need to focus on that." Use those knee-jerk reactions, along with your results from the various self-assessments in the book to figure out what you need to change—and what you don't. There's no sense in training hard to jump over a hurdle that's only an inch high. You can easily walk over that hurdle already, so you don't need to waste your time and energy on it.

In this chapter, you'll learn how to figure out which hurdles require training, and which ones don't. You'll also develop a plan for surmounting them, starting with the challenges you feel are most critical to your health and quality of life. Once you define and prioritize your survivorship goals, you'll develop a strategy—your training plan—for achieving them. You'll also develop a way to monitor your results, continually checking to see if the changes you make are actually working. If your monitoring process uncovers a flaw in your plan, you'll change direction, coming up with new strategies to try.

In this way, you put steps 1 to 6 to work for you in your life on a consistent basis. Once you do so, you'll sail over your survivorship challenges, and begin to see life from a new perspective.

PICK YOUR HURDLE

Throughout this book, you've learned numerous strategies for improving your life after cancer.

In chapter 1, you discovered how to evaluate your health-care team, things about health you should watch out for and other aspects of your overall health-care plan for getting the best care you can. In chapter 2, you learned how to educate yourself about tests, treatments, and medications in order to more effectively make health-care decisions. In subsequent chapters, you found out how to improve your communication skills, strengthen your support network, change lifestyle habits, and deal with emotional issues. That's a lot of information! Don't let it overwhelm you. You need not incorporate it all into your life at once. In fact, you shouldn't. Trying to digest and implement all of the advice you've read in the previous pages can only increase your stress even more.

So don't overload yourself with too much training. You need not circle the track of life in record time. Rather, focus on just one hurdle at a time. If you don't have a health-care team in place—or don't feel comfortable with your current set of doctors—you might start with the strategies outlined in chapter 1 first. If you feel out of touch with family and friends, you might skip the first few chapters and start your survivorship journey with chapter 4 instead. You see, although the program flows in a logical step-by-step format, none of the steps of the program require prerequisite course work. You can start your journey with any step and even skip some steps if you find you don't need them.

So how do you determine where to start? In each chapter of this book, I included self-assessments for you. Use them. They will help you to see just how well you are doing. For example, in chapter 1, you found a form to fill out to help you decide whether you were getting quality care. If you answered yes to all or most of the questions, you've got a strong health-care team in place and need not make any changes in that area. So, simply move onto step 2—becoming a more health-savvy survivor. If you find you pass the self-assessments in a given chapter, think of it as a head start on your journey around the track. You already have the right tools in place. Just move on to the next step.

What if, based on your self-assessments, you find you need to address multiple areas in your life? To further help define your goals, think about the following question:

"What do I want to change?"

For example, if you feel pain on a regular basis, you might want to start with that problem first. If you feel frustrated by your relationship with your doctor, start there. If you feel strained relationships with your family and friends, mending them and setting up a stronger support team for yourself may be the place to start. Of course, you may really want to change *numerous* things, but consider what's most important for you at this time. What emotions, symptoms, and life challenges immediately come to mind as hurdles to better health and quality of life? Again, look over your results from the various self-assessments that you took throughout this book. Your answers will help you to get a better handle on which problems need immediate attention, and which ones can safely wait a while.

Also, consider enlisting the help of a few "coaches." Ask one or two loved ones, your doctor, or spiritual advisor (whomever you feel most comfortable talking to about these issues) for help in refining your goals. Quite often, it's hard to see ourselves clearly. We easily get hung up on whatever is bothering us most on that day, at that moment. It can sometimes be hard to see the big picture. Because of this, a close friend or family member can help provide perspective. For example, let's say you *think* you want to deal with a problem at work, because about an hour ago you had a confrontation with your boss. When you mention this to your "coach," however, he or she might tell you that generally, your day-to-day and week-to-week work doesn't seem to bother you that much. Your coach might instead suggest you mend a friendship that went sour during your battle with cancer because, on a daily basis, you mention your sadness over this situation.

Once you take the self-assessments, listen to the advice of your coach, and think about what you want to change, pick a challenge to start your journey. Once you have your sights on your hurdle, then it's time to come up with the training plan you will use to clear it.

DRAW UP YOUR TRAINING PLAN

ONCE YOU KNOW your goal, it's time to come up with a plan to achieve it. To do so, use the decision-making tool that you learned in chapter 2 (see page 33). Brainstorm numerous ways to surmount your hurdle, and then pick one to follow.

For example, let's say you decided that, above all else, you need to focus on improving your emotional health first. Using the decision-making tool in chapter 2, you'd gather information about your problem. In this case, you might reread chapter 6, make an appointment with your family doctor to discuss your options, and do a Medline search to see if any new studies have uncovered novel approaches to boosting mood. Based on the information you'd have uncovered, you'd then develop a few possible plans to solve the problem. These plans might include trying medication, using bright-light therapy that you read about on Medline, or trying the thought reframing technique you learned in chapter 6. You'd then narrow these

Overcoming Planners' Block

HAVING TROUBLE COMING up with a plan to surmount your hurdle? You may have planners' block. Fear or another negative emotion may be preventing you from seeing solutions that are right in front of you. To overcome planners' block, try these strategies.

- Remember that new ideas are a combination of what you already know, fit together in new ways. Reading a book, taking a walk, or experiencing something new can be a catalyst for combining these bits of knowledge in a new way to solve a problem or think differently about a problem or challenge.
- Stop trying to formulate your plan, take a break, and return to the process later. Doing some simple task, such as taking a shower or washing dishes or driving your car, can distract your brain from the problem you are trying solve long enough to allow you to make new creative connections.
- Try to overcome your knee-jerk instinct to rule out possible solutions. Our brains are hardwired to judge ideas at the same time as we generate them, so we can respond quickly in an emergency. Yet, when you quickly rule out a possible solution by thinking, "I've been there, done that," you may lose the best solution of all.
- Consider all of your options carefully. Unfortunately, school systems teach children that there is only one right answer. Clearly, this is not true. Especially in cancer survivorship, you have the option of taking many different routes to a solution.
- Rather than trying to generate the best overall solution, focus on developing two to three possibilities. This will help to open your

plans down to just one to try. You'd implement it and then monitor your mood to see if it's working.

Of course, that's all easier said than done. You will find a vast array of ways to get in the shape you need to clear your hurdle. Which strategy will work best for you? Consider the following questions:

- *What plan do you feel most comfortable implementing?* If, like me, you generally don't like to take medication because you worry about possible side effects, then that probably isn't the best solution to your problem. On the other hand, if you're really busy and could use some time to yourself, the relaxation exercise in chapter 6 might work best.
- *What plan does your place of residence, family situation, work situation, and lifestyle most support?* Let's say you want to get in shape but live in Seattle, Washington, or Portland, Oregon, where it rains more often than it doesn't. Then an outdoor walking program may not offer the best option for you. On the other hand, joining a gym and signing up for a few sessions with a personal trainer may be the best way for you to go.
- *What plan does your coach think will work best?* Again, your trusted coach may see some aspects of your life differently than you do and be able to offer some helpful insight in narrowing down your options.

Once you pick a plan, then take a deep breath, let it out with a sigh, and relax. Try not to get hung up on developing the perfect plan right out of the block. Just as a track runner may need to occasionally tweak his or her training regimen to see better results, you, too, may need to tweak your plan. If your plan isn't perfect, that doesn't make you a failure. The only bad plan is the plan you were too scared to try. If the plan doesn't work out, you can always scrap it and try a different approach. So, now, with your plan in place, let's take a look at how you will monitor your progress to ensure that your plan is the best plan for you.

TEST YOUR PLAN

ONCE YOU KNOW what you want to change and how you plan to do it, you'll need to come up with a way to monitor your progress. Think of this monitoring process as a periodic trial that you run to see if all of your hard training is truly paying off. During your trial you might trip over your hurdle. If that's the case, you'll simply get back up, return to the start line, adjust some aspect of your plan, and then try again. On the other hand, you might find that you sail over your hurdle without a problem. If that's the case, you'll give yourself a pat on the back and move on to your next hurdle.

How do you monitor your progress? That depends on both your hurdle and the plan you're using to surmount it. Here are some possible ways to monitor your progress based on different goals:

Goal: Weight loss
Way to monitor it: Step on the scale today, record that weight, and then monitor your weight weekly.

Goal: Eat a more healthful diet
Way to monitor it: Keep a daily food log, jotting down the foods and beverages you eat and drink each day and then reviewing that log once a week to see how well you are sticking to your nutritional goals.

Goal: Reduce the frequency or severity of headaches or some other symptom
Way to monitor it: Rank the severity (how bad it is), duration (how long it lasts), and frequency (how often) of bothersome symptoms. Rank your initial symptom on a scale of 0 to 10 (using the sample symptom-rating scale on page 20) and then complete this process once or twice a day, again looking over your results once a week to see if your changes are making an impact.

Goal: Closer relationships with family members
Way to monitor it: Rank how you feel about these relationships on a scale of 1 to 10, with 1 being completely out of touch and 10 being the closest you've ever been. Ask your family members to do the same. After a few weeks, rank your intimacy level again to see if it has improved.

Goal: Lower cholesterol
Way to monitor it: Ask your doctor to run a blood panel. After a few months, get a follow-up panel completed to see if your numbers have improved. You can do the same with blood pressure and blood sugar levels.

Goal: Reduce your level of stress at work
Way to monitor it: When you arrive at work, at midday, and right before you leave for home, rank your level of stress on a scale from 0 to 10, with 0 being no stress and 10 being the worst stress you could ever feel. Keep these rankings for a few weeks and then look over your scores to see if there's a trend.

Goal: Improve your research skills
Way to monitor it: Keep a computer file or notebook that contains all the information on a topic you are researching. After looking over that information, answer this question: Do I have studies that support a realistic option or options for me to try? If so, list the options and talk to your doctor about them. If not, describe or refine your question again and keep searching.

Goal: Improve your organizational skills
Way to monitor it: Keep a diary listing the things you need to do in a given day, week, and month, or add them in a to-do list, checking them off when they are done. As you get better at this type of planning and tracking, see if the number of completed tasks are being checked off more often than in the past. Not only will this help you monitor your efficiency—how well you tackle your to-do list—but it will also help you keep tabs on your ability to plan the right number of tasks in a given period of time.

Goal: Improve your relationships with co-workers
Way to monitor it: Use a small notebook and list which colleagues you would like to reconnect with at work. Choose one person at a time. Once you develop a relationship with one person, check that person off the list and move on to the next.

Goal: Improve your level of communication with your doctor
Way to monitor it: After a visit, evaluate quickly how things went using a simple scale from 0 to 10, with 0 being not good at all to 10 being the best score you could give. Do this after each visit to see if your scores improve.

This type of self-monitoring will help you to see in black and white if your changes are truly making an impact. It will give you a clear idea of whether you are getting better, getting worse, or staying the same. It ensures that you don't just aimlessly try remedy after remedy, never really getting a sense which is working. Although this may seem like common sense, I can tell you that few survivors actually do it. I've met many survivors, who are taking numerous different pain medications, for example—yet they are still in pain. When I ask them why they are taking medications that don't work, they tell me that they take them because

SAMPLE SELF-MONITORING FORM

MONTH: April

GOAL: Reduce Fatigue

Rating		1	2	3	4	5	6	7	8	9	10	11	12	13	14	15	16	17	18	19	20	21	22	23	24	25	26	27	28	29	30	31
Worst	10																															
	9	A	A							B	B														B	B	B	B	B	B	B	B
	8			A																							B	B	B	B	B	B
	7				A	A	A	A				A	A		B										B	B						
Rating	6								A					A		B	B							B								
Scale	5																	B	B	B			B	B								
	4																				B	B										
	3																															
	2																															
	1																															
None	0																															

Days

Notes: A: Go to bed at 10:00 PM and do not stay up working late. B: I started walking half a mile after dinner.

SAMPLE SELF-MONITORING FORM

MONTH: April

GOAL: Reduce Fatigue

	1	2	3	4	5	6	7	8	9	10	11	12	13	14	15	16	17	18	19	20	21	22	23	24	25	26	27	28	29	30	31
Worst 10																															
9																															
8																															
7																															
Rating 6																															
Scale 5																															
4																															
3																															
2																															
1																															
None 0																															

Days

Notes: _____

their doctors told them to. When I ask them, "When is the last time you saw your doctor?" they often tell me it was a few years ago! A simple self-monitoring form and a follow-up visit to the doctor could probably have put all of them on the right track, and help them reduce the pain they feel.

Let's get started. You now have a goal in hand and you've come up with a plan to get there. Then either use the self-monitoring form on page 170—or some other self-monitoring method—to track your progress. On this form, 0 stands for no symptoms or behavior you want to change, and 10 means the maximum. You can use this scale for anything you want to change, just use 0 to mean the absence of the behavior/symptom and 10 to mean the worst you ever experienced with that behavior or symptom. For example, you could use this form to track fatigue, pain, anxiety, weight, exercise, or food choice. Use these pointers.

- Rate the severity or frequency (how often per day) of your symptom or the target you want to change daily at the same time each day. For example, if you are tracking your energy level, rate your level of energy at about the same time using the 0 to 10 rating scale, with 0 being no energy, 5 being an average amount of energy, and 10 being lots of energy. Remember, you can use any level between 0 and 10. Place an *A* in the square indicating your level of energy for that day. The *A* is your code for the first approach you try to improve your energy (for example, slowing down your work pace).
- Continue, each day recording your symptom or the behavior you are working on changing using your self-monitoring form. Give the approach you are trying to improve things a fair chance to work, at least for a month or so.
- After about two to three weeks, read through your self-monitoring form and see if things are improving at all. Are you feeling more energetic than when you first started, about the same, or more tired?
- If, after three to four weeks of tracking your results, you do not notice a change, keep going with the approach, but fine-tune it. For example, if you are trying to improve your energy level beyond your initial levels, and it is going slowly or not improving at all, you might also think about changing the time you are going to bed, or starting an exercise plan.
- In that case, place a *B* on the self-monitoring form to indicate that you are now trying another approach. Try this and then reassess how your energy levels are doing. If you need to readjust your program again

after you give it another two to three weeks, do so. This trial-and-error approach can really help you figure out what will best work for you. Work with your doctor, support person, or health-care provider to find the right solutions to your problem and evaluate for yourself whether it is really helping.

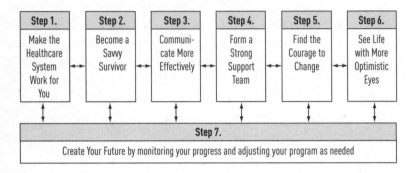

THE JOURNEY OF A LIFETIME

WHAT DO YOU do once you've cleared all of the hurdles that you set out for yourself? Well, think back to the image of that track again. It's a circle, one with no definable end. This circle represents your life after cancer. You will continue to run—or walk—around this track of life, over and over and over again. Occasionally you'll encounter more hurdles. Each time you do so, you'll employ the skills you've now learned to overcome those hurdles and move on down your path to life.

Eventually, as you do this over and over again, each hurdle will feel less and less difficult to jump. The process will become second nature to you, and you'll sail over your hurdles without really thinking about it. Once this begins to happen, you will have become what I like to call a "thriver." You will not just have survived cancer. You will not have just learned to live with your new "normal." No, you will have *created* your new normal. You will have built a new life, and possibly a better life.

Just over 73 percent of cancer survivors report at least one positive consequence of their cancer experience, and 76 percent say that cancer actually *improved* their lives. These survivors say they are better able to appreciate the small things in life, are less concerned with trivial matters, are more focused on their priorities, have become more spiritual, practice a healthier lifestyle, feel more in love with their partner, and are better socially adjusted than before their diagnosis. So it's not only possible, the statistics are in your favor. You can do this. You can surmount the challenges that stand in your way and enter a new stage of life. You can move beyond your new normal and into your new life. It's there waiting for you. Live it!

SELECTED BIBLIOGRAPHY

CHAPTER 1

Committee on Quality of Health Care in America. *Crossing the Quality Chasm: A New Health System for the 21st Century.* Washington, D.C.: Institute of Medicine/National Academy Press, 2001.

Fontana, S. A., L. C. Baumann, C. Helberg, and R. R. Love. "The Delivery of Preventive Services in Primary Care Practices According to Chronic Disease Status." *American Journal of Public Health* 87, no. 7 (1997): 1,190–6.

Jaen, C. R., K. C. Stange, and P. A. Nutting. "Competing Demands of Primary Care: A Model for the Delivery of Clinical Preventive Services." *Journal of Family Practice* 38, no. 2 (1994): 166–71.

Kohn, L., J. M. Corrigan, and M. S. Donaldson, eds. *To Err Is Human: Building a Safer Health System.* Committee on Quality of Health Care in America, Institute of Medicine, 2000.

Leape L. L., A. G. Lawthers, T. A. Brennan, and W. G. Johnson. "Preventing Medical Injury." *Quality Review Bulletin* 19, no. 5 (May 1993): 144–9.

Lewis, C. "The Impact of Direct-to-consumer Advertising." *FDA Consumer* 37, no. 2 (2003): 8.

Schommer, J., W. R. Doucetee, and B.H. Mehta. "Rote Learning after Exposure to Direct-to-Consumer Television Advertisement for a Prescription Drug." *Clinical Therapeutics* 20, no. 3 (1998): 617–32.

Snyderman, R., and R. S. Williams. "Prospective Medicine: The Next Health Care Transformation." *Academic Medicine* 78, no. 11 (2003): 1,079–84.

Wen, M., C. R. Browning, and K. A. Cagney. "Poverty, Affluence, and Income Inequality: Neighborhood Economic Structure and its Implications for Health." *Social Science and Medicine* 57 (2003): 843–60.

Wynia, M. K., J. B. VanGeest, D. S. Cummins, and I. B. Wilson. "Do Physicians Not Offer Useful Services Because of Coverage Restrictions?" *Health Affairs* 22 , no. 4 (2003): 190–7.

CHAPTER 2

Ahlberg, K., T. Ekman, F. Gaston-Johansson, and V. Mock. "Assessment and Management of Cancer-related Fatigue in Adults." *The Lancet* 362 (2003): 640–50.

Bodenheimer, T., E. H. Wagner, and K. Grumbach. "Improving Primary Care for Patients with Chronic Illness." *Journal of the American Medical Association* 288, no. 14 (2002): 1,775–9.

Bodenheimer, T., E. H., Wagner, and K. Grumback. "Improving Primary Care for Patients with Chronic Illness: The Chronic Care Model, Part 2." *Journal of the American Medical Association* 288, no. 15 (2002): 1,909–14.

Courneya, J. S., J. R. Mackey, G. J. Bell, L. W. Jones, C. J. Field, and A. S. Fairey. "Randomized Controlled Trial of Exercise Training in Postmenopausal Breast Cancer Survivors: Cardiopulmonary and Quality of Life Outcomes." *Journal of Clinical Oncology* 21, no. 9 (2003): 1,660–8.

Earle, C. C., and B. A. Neville. "Under Use of Necessary Care Among Cancer Survivors." *Cancer* 101, no. 8 (2004): 1,712–9.

Earle, C. C., H. J. Burstein, E. P. Winer, and J. C. Weeks. "Quality of Non-Breast Cancer Health Maintenance Among Elderly Breast Cancer Survivors." *Journal of Clinical Oncology* 21, no. 8 (2003): 1,447–51.

Eisenberg, D. M. "Advising Patients Who Seek Alternative Medical Therapies." *Annals of Internal Medicine* 127 (1997): 61–69.

Fellowes, D., K. Barnes, and S. Wilkinson. "Aromatherapy and massage for Symptom Relief in Patients with Cancer" (Cochrane Review) *The Cochrane Library,* issue 2. Chichester, UK: John Wiley & Sons, Ltd., 2005.

Owen, J. E., J. C. Klapow, D. L. Roth, and D. C. Tucker. "Use of the Internet for Information and Support: Disclosure Among Persons with Breast and Prostate Cancer." *Journal of Behavioral Medicine* 27, no. 5 (2004): 491–505.

Rothman, A. A., and E. H. Wagner. "Chronic Illness Management: What is the Role of Primary Care?" *Annals of Internal Medicine* 138, no. 3 (2003): 256–62.

Safran, D. G. "Defining the Future of Primary Care: What Can We Learn from Patients?" *Annals of Internal Medicine* 138, no. 3 (2003): 246–55.

Tattersall, R. L. "The Expert Patient: A New Approach to Chronic Disease Management for the Twenty-First Century." *Clinical Medicine* 2, no. 3 (2002): 227–9.

Von Korff, M., J. Gruman, J. Schaefer, S. Curry, and E. H. Wagner. "Collaborative Management of Chronic Illness." *Annals of Internal Medicine* 127, no. 12 (1997): 1,097–1,102.

CHAPTER 3

Anderson H., E. Espinosa, F. Lofts, M. Meehan, G. Hutchinson, N. Price, A. Heyes. "Evaluation of the Chemotherapy Patient Monitor: An Interactive Tool for Facilitating Communication Between Patients and Oncologists During the Cancer Consultation." *European Journal of Cancer Care* 10, no. 2 (2001): 115–23.

Ford, S., and A. Hall. "Communication Behaviours of Skilled and Less Skilled Oncologists: A Validation Study of the Medical Interaction Process System (MIPS)." *Patient Education & Counseling* 54, no. 3 (2004): 275–82.

Guadagnoli, E., and P. Ward. "Patient Participation in Decision-making." *Social Science & Medicine* 47, no. 3 (1998): 329–39.

Partridge A. H., S. Gelber, J. Peppercorn, E. Sampson, K. Knudsen, M. Laufer, R. Rosenberg, M. Przypyszny, A. Rein, and E. P Winer. "Web-based Survey of Fertility Issues in Young Women with Breast Cancer." *Journal of Clinical Oncology* 22, no. 20 (2004): 4,174–8,315.

Safran, D. G. "Defining the Future of Primary Care: What Can We Learn from Patients?" *Annals of Internal Medicine* 138, no. 3 (2003): 246–55.

Scheitel, S., B. Boland, P. Wollan, and M. Silverstein. "Patient-physician Agreement about Medical Diagnosis and Cardiovascular Risk Factors in the Ambulatory General Medical Examination." *Mayo Clinic Proceedings,* 71, no. 9 (1996): 1,131–7.

Von Korff, M., J. Gruman, J. Schaefer, S. Curry, and E. H. Wagner. "Collaborative Management of Chronic Illness." *Annals of Internal Medicine* 127, no. 12 (1997): 1,097–1,102.

Weitzman, P. F., and E. A. Weitzman. "Promoting Communication with Older Adults: Protocols for Resolving Interpersonal Conflicts and for Enhancing Interactions with Doctors." *Clinical Psychology Review* 23, no. 4 (2003): 523–35.

Wells, T., S. Falk, and P. Dieppe. "The Patients' Written Word: A Simple Communication Aid." *Patient Education & Counseling* 54, no. 2 (2004): 197–200.

CHAPTER 4

Berry D. L., and M. Catanzaro. "Persons with Cancer and Their Return to the Workplace." *Cancer Nursing* 15, no. 1 (1992): 40–61.

Borysenko, J. *Minding the Body, Mending the Mind.* New York, New York: Bantam, 1998.

Borysenko, J. *Fire in the Soul: A New Psychology of Spiritual Optimism.* New York, New York: Warner Books, 1994.

Burby, L. "What Do We Tell the Children?" *In Touch* 4, no. 1 (2002): 45–49.

Compas, B. E., N. L. Worsham, S. Ey, and D. C. Howell. "When Mom or Dad Has Cancer: II. Coping, Cognitive Appraisals, and Psychological Distress in Children of Cancer Patients." *Health Psychology* 15, no. 3 (1996): 167–75.

Davis Kirsch, S. E., P. A. Brandt, and F. M. Lewis. "Making the Most of the Moment: When a Child's Mother Has Breast Cancer." *Cancer Nursing* 26, no. 1 (2003): 47–54.

Helseth, S., and N. Ulfsaet. "Having a Parent with Cancer: Coping and Quality of Life of Children During Serious Illness in the Family." *Cancer Nursing* 26, no. 5 (2003): 355–62.

Feuerstein, M. "Thriving at Work." *The American Brain Tumor Association,* 31, no. 3 (2004): 6–8.

Johnstone, B., and H. H. Stonnington, eds. *Rehabilitation of Neuropsychological Disorders: A Practical Guide for Rehab Professionals.* New York: Taylor and Francis, 2001.

Mellon, S., and L.L. Northouse. "Family Survivorship and Quality of Life Following a Cancer Diagnosis." *Research in Nursing & Health* 24, (2001): 446–59.

Peterman A. H., G. Fitchett, M. J. Brady, L. Hernandez, and D. Cella. "Measuring Spiritual Well-being in People with Cancer: The Functional Assessment of Chronic Illness Therapy–Spiritual Well-Being Scale (FACIT-Sp)." *Annals of Behavioral Medicine* 24, no. 1 (2002): 49–58.

Rippentrop, E. A., E. M. Altmaier, J. J. Chen, E. M. Found, and V. J. Keffala. "The Relationship Between Religion/Spirituality and Physical Health, Mental Health, and Pain in a Chronic Pain Population." *Pain* 116, no. 3 (2005): 311–21.

Schmitz K. H., J. Holtzman, K. S. Courneya. L. C. Masse, S. Duval, and R. Kane. "Controlled Physical Activity Trials in Cancer Survivors: A Systematic Review and Meta-analysis." *Cancer Epidemiology, Biomarkers & Prevention* 14, no. 7 (2005): 1,588–95.

Spelten, E. R., J. H. Verbeek, A. L. Uitterhoeve, A. C. Ansink, J. van der Lelie, T. M. de Reijke, M. Kammeijer, J. C. de Haes, and M. A. Sprangers. "Cancer, Fatigue and the Return of Patients to Work: A Prospective Cohort Study." *European Journal of Cancer* 39, no. 11 (2003): 1,562–67.

Steiner J. F., T. A. Cavender, D. S. Main, and C. J. Bradley. "Assessing the Impact of Cancer on Work Outcomes: What Are the Research Needs?" *Cancer* 101, no. 8 (2004): 1,703–11.

Wallace, W. H., R. Anderson, and D. Baird, "Preservation of Fertility in Young Women Treated for Cancer." *Lancet Oncology* 5, no. 5 (2004): 269–70.

Welch, A. S., M. E. Wadsworth, and B. E. Compas. "Adjustment of Children and Adolescents to Parental Cancer: Parents' and Children's Perspectives." *Cancer* 77, no. 7 (1996): 1,409–18.

Wimberly, S. R., C. S. Carver, J. P. Laurenceau, S. D. Harris, and M. H. Antoni. "Perceived Partner Reactions to Diagnosis and Treatment of Breast Cancer: Impact on Psychosocial and Psychosexual Adjustment." *Journal of Consulting & Clinical Psychology* 73, no. 2 (2005): 300–311.

CHAPTER 5

———. "Does the Theory of Planned Behavior Mediate the Effects of an Oncologist's Recommendation to Exercise in Newly Diagnosed Breast Cancer Survivors? Results from a Randomized Controlled Trial." *Health Psychology* 24, no. 2 (2005): 189–97.

Albers, S. *Eating Mindfully.* Oakland, CA: New Harbinger Publications, 2003.

American Heart Association. *American Heart Association No-Fad Diet: A Personal Plan for Healthy Weight Loss.* New York, New York: Clarkson Potter, 2005.

Anderson-Hanley, C., M. L. Sherman, R. Riggs, V. B. Agocha, and B. E. Compas. "Neuropsychological Effects of Treatments for Adults with

Cancer: A Meta-analysis and Review of the Literature." *Journal of the International Neurospsychological Society* 9 (2003): 967–82.

Blanchard, C. M., M. M. Denniston, F. Baker, S. R. Ainsworth, K. S. Courneya, D. M. Hann, D. H. Gesme, D. Reding, T. Flynn, and J. S. Kennedy "Do Adults Change Their Lifestyle Behaviors after a Cancer Diagnosis?" *American Journal of Health Behavior 27* no. 3, (2003): 246–56.

Catalano, E. M. *The Chronic Pain Control Workbook.* Oakland, CA: New Harbinger Publications, 1987.

Cleeland C. S., G. J. Bennett, R. Dantzer, et al. "Are the Symptoms of Cancer and Cancer Treatment Due to a Shared Biologic Mechanism? A Cytokine-Immunologic Model of Cancer Symptoms." *Cancer* 97, no. 11 (2003): 2,919–25.

Chlebowski, R. T. "The American Cancer Society Guide for Nutrition and Physical Activity for Cancer Survivors: A Call to Action for Clinical Investigators." *CA: A Cancer Journal for Clinicians* 53, no. 5 (2003): 266–7.

Courneya, K. S., K. H. Karvinen, K. L. Campbell, R. G. Pearcey, G. Dundas, V. Capstick, and K. S. Tonkin. "Associations Among Exercise, Body Weight, and Quality of Life in a Population-Based Sample of Endometrial Cancer Survivors." *Gynecological Oncology* 97, no. 2 (2005): 422–30.

Djuric, Z., N. M. DiLaura, I. Jenkins, L. Darga, C. K. Jen, D. Mood, et al. "Combining Weight-Loss Counseling with the Weight Watchers Plan for Obese Breast Cancer Survivors." *Obesity Research* 10, no. 7 (2002): 657–65.

Feinstein, R. E., and M. S. Feinstein "Psychotherapy for health and lifestyle change." *Journal of Clinical Psychology.* 57(11) (2001): 1,263–75.

Friedenreich, C. M. "Physical Activity and Cancer Prevention: From Observational to Intervention Research." *Cancer Epidemiology Biomarkers & Prevention* 10 (2001): 287–301.

Jones, L. W., K. S. Courneya, A. S. Fairey, and J. R. Mackey. "Effects of an Oncologist's Recommendation to Exercise on Self-Reported Exercise Behavior in Newly Diagnosed Breast Cancer Survivors: A Single-Blind, Randomized Controlled Trial." *Annals of Behavioral Medicine* 28, no. 2 (2004): 105–13.

Hill, H. A., and H. Austin. "Nutrition and Endometrial Cancer." *Cancer Causes & Control* 7 (1996): 19–32.

Hootman, J. M., C. A. Macera, B. E. Ainsworth, et al. "Association Among Physical Activity Level, Cardiorespiratory Fitness, and Risk of Musculoskeletal Injury." *American Journal of Epidemiology* 154 (2001): 251–8.

Hu, F. B., M. J. Stampfer, J. E. Manson, et al. "Dietary Fat Intake and the Risk of Coronary Heart Disease in Women." *New England Journal of Medicine* 337 (1997): 1,491–9.

IARC Cancer Prevention Series. *Physical Activity, Body Weight, and Cancer.* Lyon, France: IARC Press, 2002.

Main, D. S., C. T. Nowels, T. A. Cavender, M. Etschmaier, and J. F. Steiner. "A Qualitative Study of Work and Work Return in Cancer Survivors." *Psycho-Oncology* 14, no. 11 (2005): 992–1,004.

Short, P. F., J. J. Vasey, and K. Tunceli. "Employment Pathways in a Large Cohort of Adult Cancer Survivors." *Cancer* 103, no. 6 (2005): 1,292–1,301.

Steiner, J. F., T. A. Cavender, D. S. Main, and C. J. Bradley. "Assessing the Impact of Cancer on Work Outcomes: What Are the Research Needs?" *Cancer* 101, no. 8 (2004): 1,703–11.

Tangney, C. C., J. A. Young, M. A. Murtaugh, M. A. Cobleigh, and D. M. Oleske. "Self-Reported Dietary Habits, Overall Dietary Quality and Symptomatology of Breast Cancer Survivors: A Cross-Sectional Examination." *Breast Cancer Research & Treatment* 71, no. 2 (2002): 113–23.

Yabroff, K. R., W. F. Lawrence, S. Clauser, W. W. Davis, and M. L. Brown. "Burden of Illness in Cancer Survivors: Findings from a Population-Based National Sample." *Journal of the National Cancer Institute.* 96, no. 17 (2004): 1,322–30.

Yonemoto, T., S. Tatezaki, T. Ishii, and Y. Hagiwara. "Marriage and Fertility in Long-Term Survivors of High Grade Osteosarcoma." *American Journal of Clinical Oncology* 26, no. 5 (2003): 513–6.

CHAPTER 6

Ables, A. Z., and O. L Baughman. "Antidepressants: Update on New Agents and Indications." *American Family Physician* 67, no. 3 (2003): 547–54.

Carver C. S., R. G. Smith, M. H. Antoni, V. M. Petronis, S. Weiss, and R. P. Derhagopian. "Optimistic Personality and Psychosocial Well-being During Treatment Predict Psychosocial Well-being Among Long-term Survivors of Breast Cancer. *Health Psychology* 24, no. 5 (2005): 508–16.

Davis, M., E. Robbins, and M. Mckay, *Relaxation & Stress Reduction Workbook,* 5th ed. Oakland, CA: New Harbinger Publications, 2000.

Emery, G. *Overcoming Depression.* Oakland, CA: New Harbinger Publications, 2000.

Fuller, M. A., and M. Sajatovic. *Drug Information Handbook for Psychiatry 1999–2000.* Hudson, Ohio: Lexi-Comp Inc., 1999.

Jacobsen, P. B., M. A. Andrykowski, and C. L. Thors. "Relationship of Catastrophizing to Fatigue Among Women Receiving Treatment for Breast Cancer." *Journal of Consulting & Clinical Psychology* 72, no. 2 (2004): 355–61.

McGregor, B. A., M. H. Antoni, A. Boyers, S. M. Alferi, B. B. Blomberg, and C. S. Carver. "Cognitive-Behavioral Stress Management Increases Benefit Finding and Immune Function Among Women with Early-Stage Breast Cancer." *Journal of Psychosomatic Research* 56, no. 1 (2004): 1–8.

McKenzie. H., and M. Crouch. "Discordant Feelings in the Lifeworld of Cancer Survivors." *Health* (London) 8, no. 2 (2004): 139–57.

National Cancer Institute. "Depression and Supportive Care." www.cancer .gov/cancerinfo/pdq/supportivecare/depression/HealthProfessional, accessed June 14, 2005.

Rehse, B., and R. Pukrop. "Effects of Psychosocial Interventions on Quality of Life in Adult Cancer Patients: Meta-analysis of 37 Published Controlled Outcome Studies." *Patient Education & Counseling* 50, no. 2 (2003): 179–86.

Temoshok, L. R. "Complex Coping Patterns and Their Role in Adaptation and Neuroimmunomodulation: Theory, Methodology, and Research." *Annals of the New York Academy of Sciences* 917 (2000): 446–55.

Ursano, R. J. "Post-Traumatic Stress Disorder." *New England Journal of Medicine* 346, no. 2 (2002): 130–2.

Wolff, S., C. Nichols, D. Ulman, A. Miller, S. Kho, D. Lofye, M. Milford, D. Tracy, B. Bellavia, and L. Armstrong, "Survivorship: An Unmet Need of the Patient with Cancer—Implications of a Survey of the Lance Armstrong Foundation (LAF) Abstract 6032. Presentation at the American Society of Clinical Oncologists, 2005.

Yehuda, R. "Post-Traumatic Stress Disorder." *New England Journal of Medicine* 346, no. 2 (2002): 108–14.

CHAPTER 7

Donaldson, L. "Expert Patients Usher in a New Era of Opportunity for the NHS." *British Medical Journal* 14 (2003): 1,279–80.

Groves, T., E. H. Wagner. "High Quality Care for People with Chronic Diseases." *British Medical Journal* 19 (2005): 609–10.

Lorig, K. "Partnerships Between Expert Patients and Physicians." *The Lancet* 359, no. 9, 309 (2002): 814–5.

Lorig. K, D. S. Sobel, A. L. Stewart, B. W. Brown, A. Bandura, P. Ritter, et al. "Evidence Suggesting That a Chronic Disease Self-Management Program Can Improve Health Status while Reducing Hospitalization: A Randomized Trial." *Medical Care* 37 (1999): 5–14.

Macdonald, L., J. Bruce, N. W. Scott, W. C. Smith, and W. A. Chambers. "Long-term Follow-up of Breast Cancer Survivors with Post-mastectomy Pain Syndrome." *British Journal of Cancer* 31 (2005): 225–30.

Roberts, S., C. Black, and K. Todd. "The Living with Cancer Education Programme, II. Evaluation of an Australian Education and Support Programme for Cancer Patients and Their Family and Friends." *European Journal of Cancer Care* 11, no. 4 (2002): 280–9.

Wagner, E. H, B. T. Austin, C. Davis, M. Hindmarsh, J. Schaefer, and A. Bonomi. "Improving Chronic Illness Care: Translating Evidence into Action." *Health Affairs (Millwood)* 20, no. 6 (2001): 64–78.

Resources

A T TIMES A site is included more than once within the appendix to highlight various aspects that may benefit you.

CHAPTER 1

Abramson Cancer Center of the University of Pennsylvania
www.oncolink.com
Phone: 1-800-789-PENN
Provides comprehensive cancer information for patients, families, and providers; sponsored by the University of Pennsylvania.

Cancer Care
www.cancercare.org
Phone: 1-800-813-HOPE
Provides information on ways to advocate for yourself or someone else who has cancer, on health insurance and financial issues.

The Cancer Center
www.healthsystem.virginia.edu/internet/cancer
Phone: 1-800-223-9173
Proves a comprehensive library of information about cancer, treatment, diagnosis, nutrition, and genetics. Sponsored by the University of Virginia's Cancer Care Center.

Centers for Medicare and Medicaid Services
www.cms.hhs.gov
Phone: 1-800-MEDICARE
Provides overview and assistance for issues related to Medicare and Medicaid.

Department of Health and Human Services
Centers for Disease Control and Prevention
www.cdc.gov
Phone: 1-800-CDC-INFO
Provides cancer statistics and guidelines for preventive care. It hosts many links for further information on cancer and cancer-related topics.

Health Care Information Resources
www.hsl.mcmaster.ca/tomflem/cancer.html
Phone: 1-905-525-9140 ext. 22321
This site provides a listing of health-care resource Web sites in both the United States and Canada for patients, family members, and professionals.

Institute of Medicine
www.iom.edu
Phone: 1-202-334-2352
A primary source for scientifically based information on biomedical, medical, health, and mental health information.

National Cancer Institute
U.S. National Institutes of Health
http://cancernet.nci.nih.gov
Phone: 1-800-4-CANCER
Provides scientifically based information on all aspects of cancer treatment and ongoing care. It provides a list of clinical trials and links to other informative sites.

Tricare

www.tricare.osd.mil

Provides information on the U.S. military health-care plan.

Veterans Affairs

www.va.gov

Provides information on benefits and services available to veterans.

CHAPTER 2

American Cancer Society

Cancer Survivors Network

www.acscsn.org

Phone: 1-800-ACS-2345

A site for dialogue with other cancer survivors regarding their experiences; it allows for questions and answers, chat forums, and an "Expression Gallery" where poems or other forms of self-expression can be posted.

Association of Cancer Online Resources

www.acor.org

Phone: 1-212-226-5525

This sits hosts a complication of Web links on cancer, cancer treatment, and other cancer-related topics.

Cancer Care

www.cancercare.org

Phone: 1-800-813-HOPE

Provides free professional support services, including counseling, education, financial assistance, and practical help, by trained oncology social workers, to anyone affected by cancer.

A Cancer Survivor's Compendium

www.hopeandhealing.com

Phone: Web only

Provides an extensive directory of resources for living well after cancer.

Cochrane Collaboration

www.cochrane.org
Phone: Web only
Hosts the search engine for Cochrane Collaboration studies.

National Association of Insurance Commissioners

www.naic.org
Phone: Follow Web links by state for applicable phone numbers
By state, this site allows access to local insurance commissioners for you
to contact if you find you are having difficulty with your insurance carrier
or policy.

National Association of Social Workers

www.naswdc.org
Phone: 1-202-408-8600
Source to help locate a social worker in your location.

National Center for Complementary and Alternative Medicine

http://nccam.nih.gov
Phone: 1-888-644-6226
Provides a source for locating federally funded studies on CAM.

NeedyMeds

www.needymeds.com
Phone: 1-215-625-9609 (For general questions, otherwise use Web link–
provided phone numbers for individual questions.)
This site is designed to provide information about patient-assistance
programs that provide no-cost prescription medications to eligible
participants.

PubMed

www.pubmed.org
Phone: Web only
Hosts the search engine for PubMed, allowing searches of scientific
literature.

Social Security Administration
www.ssa.gov
Phone: 1-800-772-1213
Government Web site to answer questions regarding disability benefits.

The Susan G. Komen Breast Cancer Foundation
www.komen.org
Helpline: 1-800-IM-AWARE
Provides information and support to patients, survivors, and their loved ones. Search "after treatment" for information on survivorship. Also provides information in Spanish.

PHARMACEUTICAL RESOURCES
For each of the following, search "patient assistance programs."

Merck & Co.
www.merck.com
Phone: 1-800-727-5400

GlaxoSmithKline
http://us.gsk.com/card
Phone: 1-888-ORANGE-6 (1-888-672-6436)

Pfizer
www.pfizer.com
Phone: Check Web site; numbers are associated with medications sought.

NovartisAG
www.pharma.us.novartis.com
Phone: 1-888-NOW-NOVA (1-888-669-6682)
Aventis

www.sanofi-aventis.us
Phone: 1-212-704-8242

Roche Group
www.rocheusa.com
Phone: 1-877-75ROCHE (1-877-757-6243)

CHAPTER 3

Cancer Center Report
www.usc.edu/hsc/info/pr/ccr/02spring/council.html
Phone: Web only
A link to a report that describes the Cancer Survivorship Advisory Council
guidelines to ensure that physicians interact and communicate with their
patients in a compassionate manner.

Lance Armstrong Foundation
www.livestrong.org
Phone: 1-866-235-7205
Web site of a nonprofit organization with a mission to inspire and empower
people with cancer to live strong. They serve their mission through education, advocacy, public health, and research programs. Search "take control"
for many practical tips.

The Susan G. Komen Breast Cancer Foundation
http://healthology.komen.org
Helpline: 1-800-IM-AWARE
Search "talk to your doctor."

CHAPTER 4

Lance Armstrong Foundation
www.livestrong.org
Phone: 1-866-235-7205
Web site of a nonprofit organization with a mission to inspire and empower
people with cancer to live strong. They serve their mission through education, advocacy, public health, and research programs. Search "healthy
behaviors."

Medical News Today
www.medicalnewstoday.com
Phone: Web only
Provides the latest medical news and health news in a bulleted format.

Articles covered are of scientific studies, and names and contact information are presented for readers to follow up with the individual researchers.

National Cancer Institute
http://plan2005.cancer.gov
Phone: 1-800-4-CANCER
Search site for this publication: "Cancer Survivorship: Optimizing Health and Quality of Life after Cancer"

People Living with Cancer
www.plwc.org
Phone: 1-703-299-0150
This is a patient-information Web site of the American Society of Clinical Oncology (ASCO). It is designed to help patients and their loved ones to make informed health-care decisions. The site provides information on many types of cancer, clinical trials, coping, side effects, a "Find an Oncologist" database, message boards, and patient-support organizations.

CHAPTER 5

American Cancer Society
www.cancer.org
Phone: 1-800-ACS-2345
If you were not familiar with this information, the following brief summary of the nutrition information from the American Cancer Society will help give you some overall guidance on what the experts think is a healthy diet. More detailed information, along with scientific studies that support these recommendations, is available on their Web site.

These recommendations were developed by the American Cancer Society, 2001 Nutrition and Physical Activity Guidelines Advisory Committee.

AMERICAN CANCER SOCIETY DIET (OUR SUMMARY)
1. **Eat a variety of healthful foods, with an emphasis on plant sources.**
   - *Healthful foods* means that you should try to choose whole grains rather than refined or processed grains and sugars, and limit you the amount of red meats that you eat. Also, avoid fried foods.

- *Plant sources* means you want to try to eat five or more servings of a variety of vegetables and fruits each day.

2. **Develop a physically active lifestyle.**
   - *Physically active* means that as an adult you should engage in at least moderate activity for thirty minutes or more on five or more days of the week; five minutes or more of moderate to vigorous activity on five or more days per week.

3. Keep your weight at a healthy level.
   - A *healthful weight* means that you should eat the right amount of calories to maintain a weight that is healthy for your height.
   - Watch portion sizes when you are eating at a restaurant and at home, too.

4. **Limit how much alcohol you drink.**

Further resources on diet and exercise:

Center for Disease Control
www.cdc.gov
Phone: Web only
The CDC's Nutrition and Physical Activity Web site contains information, recommendations, and publications on physical activity. Search "physical activity."

American Cancer Society
www.cancer.org
Phone: Web only
The American Cancer Society's Food and Fitness Web site contains information on becoming and staying active.Search "food and fitness."

The National Institute of Diabetes and Digestive and Kidney Diseases
www.niddk.nih.gov
Phone: Web only
Part of the National Institutes of Health (NIH), the Physical Activity and Weight Control Web site contains information, tips, and additional resources. Search "physical activity and weight control."

American College of Sports Medicine

www.acsm.org

Phone: 1-317-637-9200

Site provides national exercise guidelines as well as advice on how to purchase exercise equipment.

Brigham and Women's Hospital

http://healthgate.partners.org

Phone: 1-617-732-5500

The Web site of Brigham and Women's Hospital provides educational information on all aspects of cancer treatment and ongoing care. Search "interactive tools" for some useful tools to help your self-evaluation of your health and physical activity.

Lance Armstrong Foundation

www.livestrong.org

Phone: 1-866-235-7205

Search for resources on communicating with your partner.

INFORMATION ON PAIN MANAGEMENT

American Pain Foundation

www.painfoundation.org

Phone: 1-888-615-PAIN

Provides information on research being conducted on a variety of conditions, including cancer and treatment-related pain.

American Pain Society

www.ampainsoc.org

Phone: 1-847-375-4715

Provides information on pain treatment, but also hosts a search site for practitioners in your area.

CHAPTER 6

American Psychological Association
www.apa.org
Phone: 1-800-374-2721
Hosts a listing of psychologists in your area.

Canadian Health Network
www.canadian-health-network.ca
Phone: 1-888-939-3333
This provides information about the Canadian Health Network in both English and French. The information presented is useful to anyone who may enter the site, as most is informative about health and health care in general.

Cancer Care
www.cancercare.org
Phone: 1-800-813-HOPE
Provides free professional support services, including counseling and practical help, by trained oncology social workers, to anyone affected by cancer.

Center for Independent Living (CIL)
www.virtualcil.net/cils
Phone: Web only
Search for your individual state to find information and resources on a variety of community programs and services for those with disabilities.

Disability Info
www.disabilityinfo.gov
Phone: Web only
Provides general information on disability and the government-related programs; hosted by the federal government.

Gillette Cancer Connection for Women Living with Cancer

www.gillettecancerconnect.org

Phone: Web only

Provides fact sheets and tips on how to talk to friends, co-workers, spouses, and children about cancer and the survivor experience; sponsored by Proctor and Gamble.

Job Accommodation Network.

www.jan.wvu.edu

Phone: 1-800-526-7234

This links to an organization that facilitates the employment and retention of workers with disabilities by providing employers, employment providers, people with disabilities, their family members, and other interested parties with information on job accommodations, self-employment, small-business opportunities, and related subjects.

The National Coalition of Cancer Survivorship

www.canceradvocacy.org

Phone: 1-202- 464-5000

This is the Web site of the oldest survivor-led cancer advocacy organization in the country. It is an organization that is highly respected at the federal level, for advocating for quality cancer care for all Americans and empowering cancer survivors. Search "employment," "laws," and "job interviews."

MD Anderson Cancer Center

www.mdanderson.org

Phone: 1-800-392-1611

A Web site for the cancer care center, which also provides information on research and answers questions on many survivor topic areas.

State Worker's Compensation Board

www.dol.gov

Phone: 1-866-4-USA-DOL

Provides current policies and laws, by state, for those who are covered under worker's compensation.

The Susan G. Komen Breast Cancer Foundation Headquarters

www.breastfriends.com

Phone (Helpline): 1-800-IM-AWARE

Provides an opportunity to volunteer to help "fight for a cure" of breast cancer by becoming involved in fund-raising activities, such as races or writing letters to your congressional representatives to increase funding for research for a cure.

Team Survivor

www.teamsurvivor.org

Phone: Follow links to specific locale

A nonprofit organization that provides free physical activity, health education, and support programs for women affected by cancer.

CHAPTER 7

American Cancer Society

Cancer Survivors Network

www.acscsn.org

Phone: 1-800-ACS-2345

A site for dialogue with other cancer survivors regarding their experiences. In conjunction with the National Cancer Institute, free booklets are offered for ongoing self-management. Search "life after cancer treatment."

Brigham and Women's Hospital

http://healthgate.partners.org

Phone: 1-617-732-5500

The Web site of Brigham and Women's Hospital provides educational information on all aspects of cancer treatment and ongoing care. Search "health" and "newsletters," and "interactive tools" for some useful tools to help you self-evaluate your health.

Chronic Disease Management, Ministry of British Columbia

www.healthservices.gov.bc.ca

Phone: 1-250-952-3124

The site offers many tips and fact sheets on managing chronic illnesses. Search self-management of chronic illness.

Expert Patient Programme

www.expertpatients.nhs.uk

Phone: Individuals in the UK: check site for phone numbers by region)

This site provides and overview of the Expert Patient Programme, with links to articles and fact sheets on the self-management of several chronic illnesses.

Improving Chronic Care

A Program of the Robert Wood Johnston Foundation

www.improvingchroniccare.org

Phone: (Self-Management Support) 1-206-287-2077

(The Improving Chronic Illness Care Program): 1-206-287-2704

Provides an overview of a chronic illness care program created by the national expert, Dr. Edward Wagner. The site provides bibliographies and links to informative Web sites.

Lance Armstrong Foundation

www.livestrong.org

Phone: 1-866-235-7205

Web site of a nonprofit organization with a mission to inspire and empower people with cancer to live strong. They serve their mission through education, advocacy, public health, and research programs. Search "survivor tools" and "LIVESTRONG SurvivorCare Program."

APPENDIX B

Not All Medication Is the Same

DRUG	AVAILABILITY	DISORDERS	SIDE EFFECTS*
TRICYCLIC ANTIDEPRESSANTS (TCAs)			Cardiac arrhythmias, weight gain
Elavil (amitriptyline)	Tablets, injection*	Depression, chronic pain*	Marked sedation, dizziness, headache, weight gain
Anafranil (clomipramine)	Capsules*	Depression, chronic pain, panic attacks, OCD*	Dizziness, drowsiness, headache, weight gain
Norpramin (desipramine)	Tablets*	Depression, chronic pain*	Mild sedation, increased appetite, nausea
Sinequan (doxepin)	Capsules*	Depression, anxiety*	Moderate to severe sedation, dizziness, headache, weight gain
Tofranil (imipramine)	Capsules, tablets, injection*	Depression, chronic pain, panic disorder*	Moderate to severe sedation, dizziness, headache, weight gain, sexual side effects

DRUG	AVAILABILITY	DISORDERS	SIDE EFFECTS*
Pamelor (nortriptyline)	Capsules, oral solution*	Depression, chronic pain*	Mild sedation, constipation, nausea, increased appetite
SELECTIVE SEROTONIN REUPTAKE INHIBITORS (SSRIs)			Few cardiovascular adverse effects but some sexual dysfunction
Celexa (citalopram)	Tablets, oral solution®	Depression®	Sexual dysfunction, insomnia, dry mouth, nausea
Prozac (fluoxetine)	Capsules, tablets, oral solution®	Depression, OCD, bulimia nervosa®	Anxiety, nervousness, insomnia, weight loss (in cancer patients), sexual dysfunction
Luvox (fluvoxamine)	Tablets®	OCD, Depression®	Nausea, sexual dysfunction, headache, nervousness, insomnia, drowsiness
Paxil (paroxetine)	Tablets, oral suspension®	Depression, panic disorder, OCD, social phobia, GAD, PTSD®	Anxiety, nervousness, insomnia, mild weight loss (in cancer patients), headache, sexual dysfunction
Zoloft (sertraline)	Tablets, oral concentrate®	Depression, panic disorder, OCD, PTSD, PMDD®	Anxiety, nervousness, insomnia, weight loss, headache, sexual dysfunction
MONOAMINE OXIDASE INHIBITORS (MAOIs)			
Parnate (tranylcypromine)	Tablets*	Depression*	Drowsiness, hyperexcitability, headache

DRUG	AVAILABILITY	DISORDERS	SIDE EFFECTS*
Nardil (phenelzine)	Tablets*	Depression*	Drowsiness, hyperexcitability, headache
ATYPICAL ANTIDEPRESSANTS			
Wellbutrin (bupropion)	Tablets*	Depression, smoking cessation*	Agitation, insomnia, headache, confusion, dizziness, seizures, weight loss
Desyrel (trazodone)	Tablets*	Depression*	Mild sedation, dizziness, headache, confusion, muscle tremors
Serzone (nefazodone)	Tablets*	Depression, PTSD*	Headache, drowsiness, insomnia, agitation, confusion, nausea, tremors
Remeron (mirtazapine)	Tablets®	Depression®	Dizziness, increased appetite and weight gain, constipation, confusion
Effexor (venlafaxine)	Tablets, capsules®	Depression, GAD®	Headache, dizziness, insomnia, nausea, constipation, abnormal ejaculation
PSYCHOSTIMULANTS			Can be used to reverse pain killer sedative effects
Dexedrine (dextroamphetamine)	Tablets, capsules*	Exogenous obesity, ADHD*	Drug tolerance, abuse, and dependency possible, nervousness, restlessness, insomnia

DRUG	AVAILABILITY	DISORDERS	SIDE EFFECTS*
Ritalin (methylphenidate)	Tablets*	ADHD*	Drug tolerance, abuse, and dependency possible, nervousness, insomnia, anorexia, drowsiness, dizziness

* Fuller, M.A., M. Sajatovic. *Drug Information Handbook for Psychiatry 1999–2000.* Hudson, Ohio: Lexi-Comp Inc., 1999.

® Ables, A.Z., O.L.Baughman. "Antidepressants: Update on New Agents and Indications." *American Family Physician* 67, no. 3 (2003): 547–54.

National Cancer Institute. "Depression and Supportive Care." (2004) www.cancer.gov/cancerinfo/pdq/supportivecare/depression/HealthProfessional

INDEX